Nursing Knowledge

For the nurses and scholars who have influenced me.

Constance Risjord

Norman Risjord

Arleen Winter

Nursing Knowledge

Science, Practice, and Philosophy

Mark Risjord

Philosophy Department and
The Nell Hodgson Woodruff School of Nursing
Emory University

WILEY-BLACKWELL

A John Wiley & Sons, Ltd., Publication

Blackwell Publishing was acquired by John Wiley & Sons in February 2007. Blackwell's publishing programme has been merged with Wiley's global Scientific, Technical, and Medical business to form Wiley-Blackwell.

Registered office:
John Wiley & Sons Ltd, The Atrium, Southern Gate, Chichester, West Sussex, PO19 8SQ, United Kingdom

Editorial offices:
9600 Garsington Road, Oxford, OX4 2DQ, United Kingdom
2121 State Avenue, Ames, Iowa 50014-8300, USA

For details of our global editorial offices, for customer services and for information about how to apply for permission to reuse the copyright material in this book please see our website at www.wiley.com/wiley-blackwell.

Library of Congress Cataloging-in-Publication Data

Risjord, Mark W., 1960-
    Nursing knowledge : science, practice, and philosophy / Mark Risjord.
        p. ; cm.
    Includes bibliographical references and index.
    ISBN 978-1-4051-8434-2 (pbk. : alk. paper)
    1. Nursing–Philosophy.   2. Nursing–Practice.   I. Title.
    [DNLM: 1. Nursing Theory.   2. Health Knowledge, Attitudes, Practice.
3. Nursing Process.   4. Philosophy, Nursing. WY 86 R595n 2010]
    RT84.5.R57 2010
    610.73–dc22

                                                                2009020260

A catalogue record for this book is available from the British Library.

Set in 10/12pt Palatino by Aptara® Inc., New Delhi, India
Printed and bound in Malaysia by KHL Printing Co Sdn Bhd

1   2010

Contents

Preface

My intellectual engagement with nursing began with a question about teaching. The Nell Hodgson Woodruff School of Nursing at Emory University had just created a PhD program, and Professors Sandra Dunbar and Margret Moloney were teaching "the theory course." They called to ask for advice about readings in the philosophy of science. I was at a bit of a loss. Like many philosophers of science, I thought that philosophy of science should connect directly with the sciences. Only when the problems are understood from the perspective of the scientists can the important questions be asked. Since I had no understanding of nursing research, I had no clue about how to answer their simple question about a reading list.

The solution, which the Nursing School was happy to support, was to have me coteach the course. Working with PhD-level students would provide a sense of the philosophical questions that arose from nursing research. My intention was to find some philosophically and pedagogically useful readings for the course, and then return to the quiet life of a philosopher. I found, to my delight, a new world for philosophical reflection. Nurse scholars had been writing about philosophical issues for almost 40 years. While philosophers had not paid attention to them, they had been paying attention to us. The philosophical issues were clearly recognizable, and the context of nursing research and practice gave them a fresh aspect. I have taught, cotaught, or lectured in this course every year since its inception, and it remains some of the most rewarding teaching I do.

After several years of teaching the course, I began to kick around ideas for a book that would systematically treat the philosophical issues in nursing science. It was the fall semester of 2006 when a student question catalyzed the ideas. We were wrapping up our discussion of values in science. The students had worked through Longino, Harding, and other feminist philosophers of science. This is all very interesting, they said, but what does it have to do with *nursing* science? In the ensuing conversation, I was struck by the analogy between nursing roles and the oppressed social roles that give rise to epistemic standpoints. With the idea of a nursing standpoint, serious work on this book began.

The phrase "nursing knowledge" is ambiguous. It might plausibly refer to knowledge that individual nurses gain through their training and experience. While the topic is vitally important, this book will not be directly concerned with the knowledge that goes into the decisions or care plans of the practicing nurse. Rather, we will be concerned with the kind of knowledge on which the nursing profession is based. This knowledge is developed within the research enterprise of nursing, maintained in the academy, and transmitted through professional publications. Ultimately, of course, the two senses should join: the knowledge of individual nurses should be informed by disciplinary knowledge. When disciplinary knowledge does not support professional nursing, a theory–practice gap emerges.

This work will bring ideas and arguments from the philosophy of science to the discussion of nursing theory. The object is *not* to create a new nursing theory. Nor will there be sustained evaluation of, or commentary on, nursing theories. Rather, we will engage what could be called nursing "metatheory," that is, theory about theory. Since the late 1950s, nursing has had lively debates about what forms theory should take, about the unity of the discipline, about the status of borrowed theory, and so on. These debates have been philosophical, and have drawn on philosophical writings, but they have been debates among nurse scholars. In keeping with the idea that the philosophy of science ought to be rooted in philosophical questions arising from scientific practice, this work will primarily engage with the nursing metatheoretical literature. It will elucidate the historical and contemporary nursing debates and critically evaluate the arguments. While we will develop ideas within the philosophy of science, the primary audience of this work is not philosophers, but nurse scholars.

A book with two audiences risks leaving both unsatisfied. If the technical details are passed over, philosophers may find the arguments superficial. If presented in all of their abstract glory, nurse scholars may find the arguments pedantic. This problem is partly addressed below by the chapter divisions. Some chapters (5, 8, 10, 14, and 17) are devoted mostly to philosophical positions, arguments, and counter-arguments. Readers who want to understand the full philosophical background to the ideas developed in the other parts of the book will need to work through these chapters. Those who are familiar with the philosophy of science, and who are primarily interested in the ramifications of postpositivist philosophy of science for nursing, might skip them. Those readers interested in an overview of the position developed in this book might read the introduction to each Part and Chapters 3, 7, 12, and 19.

This book is the culmination of 10 years of thought about nursing science. The nurse scholars who patiently taught me about their discipline have my deep admiration and sincere appreciation: Sandra Dunbar, Margret Moloney, Kenneth Hepburn, Sue Donaldson, and every one of the nursing doctoral students who have come through Emory's program. During this period, my thinking about theory and methodology was sharpened by some very special colleagues in the humanities and the social sciences. I hope that Ivan Karp, Cory Kratz, Martine Brownley, Kareem

Khalifa, and Robert McCauley see something of themselves reflected in this work. A number of colleagues read and commented on this book at various phases of completion. Feedback of this sort is invaluable and I am deeply grateful to Ulf Nilsson, John Paley, Emily Parker, Norman Risjord, Stephanie Solomon, Alison Wylie, and especially Beverly Whelton for their thoughtful responses. Finally, this book was entirely written during my tenure as Associate Dean of the Graduate School. It would have been impossible but for the support of Dean Lisa Tedesco. She not only helped me find the balance between research and administration, but she also made substantive contributions to my thinking about these issues.

Special appreciation must be reserved for Barbara, Andrea, and Hannah Risjord. Throughout the process of writing this book, they supported me in uncountable ways and suffered both my absences and absentmindedness.

Foreword

Nursing Knowledge is a unique and compelling contribution to the body of philosophical work in nursing. Mark Risjord offers a fresh perspective of the evolution of nursing theory, science, and practice as seen through the lens of a philosopher. Risjord comprehensively analyzes the history of the development of the professional discipline of nursing. He includes all the major threads of philosophical thought, identifying their origins, critical differences, and potential for primacy. By revealing the historical juxtaposition of competing philosophies of nursing, he retraces nursing's tortuous path and conveys the passion of its scholars for the discipline and the practice. But this book is not a dry text; it reads as an exciting documentary that relates the development of nursing philosophy in the context of an evolving professional practice of nursing and an evolving general philosophy of science. Risjord goes beyond analysis of the writings to consider the philosophical debates in nursing in the context of societal changes in the status of women and nurses in health care along with the continuous transformation of philosophy of science into successive postpositivist forms. Each philosophical thread in nursing is addressed, treated as valid, and appropriately placed in the evolution of contemporary philosophy of nursing. But there are some surprising revelations from Risjord's philosophical analysis.

A major advance in this book comes from Risjord's presentation of disparate views as valuable to the evolution of nursing knowledge and science rather than as distractions. Risjord documents that while philosophers of nursing strived for consensus and adoption of a single model to unify the discipline; opposing views were key to clarifying the purpose of the discipline and developing its knowledge. A notable and valuable contribution to nursing philosophy is Risjord's analysis of the pervasive impact of logical positivism over time, despite nursing's rejection of this philosophy of science. One becomes aware of Risjord's prowess as a philosopher in his analysis of the subtle and, apparently, unrecognized influence of positivism, even in recent presentations and publications of philosophers in nursing. I had not recognized this evidence and thus was surprised by his findings. It is extremely important for nursing to fully understand the philosophical underpinnings of its models for knowledge and theory generation and this book teaches by example how this is done. Risjord offers an alternate, nonpositivist, conceptual model for generating value-laden theory to assist nursing in its quest for scientific discovery that is relevant to nursing practice and to the understanding of human health in general.

Risjord captures the prevailing sense of urgency on the part of nurse scholars to articulate a unique and defining conceptual model or grand theory of nursing. Identification of a unique discipline and science of nursing was and still continues to be needed to respond to external threats to the legitimacy of nursing as a profession and as a field of PhD study. Internally, nursing scholars fiercely and legitimately debated the directionality of influence of practice and knowledge. For the beginning scholar or student in nursing, this book is an essential companion to the reading of original classic and contemporary philosophical papers in nursing because it clarifies the unique contribution and historical context of each. This book is a definitive guide to the universe of nursing knowledge and philosophy. For the seasoned scholar, *Nursing Knowledge* reads as a compelling documentary that recasts long-standing debates on the nature and generation of nursing knowledge in a new mode and revisits the relationship of theory to practice. *Nursing Knowledge* takes the reader on an historical trip that celebrates disparate views on philosophical issues as a natural part of the evolution of the discipline and its relationship to the practice of nursing. What is unexpected is the progressive philosophy of nursing that awaits the reader at journey's end. Risjord does not disappoint; he transports the reader into a new frame of reference, a new philosophy, for advancing nursing knowledge in a manner that promises to make it more relevant to practice and theoretically coherent.

In his analysis of philosophy of nursing science, Risjord focuses on nursing's continuing utilization of hierarchical disciplinary structures, such as metaparadigm/paradigm and grand/middle-range/situation theory. This analysis alone makes the book required reading. He points out that while these structures serve the purpose of identifying a unique domain of nursing knowledge, they are at odds with nursing's professed preference for postpositivist philosophical views of value-laden science, including nursing's intent to bridge the theory–practice gap. Risjord argues that hierarchical structures isolate nursing knowledge from that of other disciplines, thus limiting the impact of nursing in advancing an enlightened view of human health across disciplines. His analysis of the separation of qualitative and quantitative research into distinct paradigms within the discipline is particularly astute; it reveals that, while intellectually convenient, this separation limits the overall support for critical theories in nursing. Perhaps the most shocking of his revelations is that hierarchical disciplinary structures in nursing emanate from the positivist viewpoint.

As an alternate, Risjord offers a radically different, nonpositivist philosophical view of knowledge structure that was first introduced by Quine ([1953] 1961). In this frame of reference, human knowledge is viewed as an integrated whole of theories from many disciplines; individual disciplines influence the whole of knowledge to the extent that their theories are coherent with those of other disciplines. Disciplines are expected to work within a unique perspective and to offer theories that reflect this perspective; but the ultimate goal is to find external support for the theories of the discipline of origin. Risjord presents this model of theory coherence in a distinctive and memorable way using the metaphors of a quilt and a spider web. Theories are depicted as nodes of a spider web that gain structural support and utility based on coherent linkages to other theories, irrespective of discipline of origin. Risjord makes a strong case for seeking coherence of theories originating in nursing across many disciplines. In the coherence model, nursing is free to link its theories to those in other fields to gain to support for them and to offer theoretical support for theories beyond nursing. The theory coherence model offers nursing a more expansive means of generating knowledge to advance the values and practice of the profession. Within a coherence framework, nursing has the potential to develop knowledge for the world as well as the practice of nursing. As a relatively young discipline, nursing is justified in considering the possibility of losing its disciplinary identity through interdisciplinary research. In Risjord's conceptualization of theory coherence, nursing practice unifies the discipline, allowing nursing to share theory and knowledge. Supportive linkages to other disciplines can be created without losing nursing's distinctive disciplinary perspective. In turn, nursing can use theory from other sources not for the purpose of "borrowing" but rather for establishing coherence and support for nursing theories.

Risjord makes a compelling case for restructuring nursing knowledge into a model that is theoretically coherent and practically relevant. Most importantly, he offers a new philosophy of nursing to guide its knowledge development. *Nursing Knowledge* is essential reading, not just to trace the evolution of nursing science and knowledge, but to frame the philosophical issues for the next round of scholarly debates and to position nursing for a transdisciplinary role in knowledge development.

Sue K. Donaldson, PhD, RN, FAAN
Distinguished Professor of Nursing and Interdisciplinary Science
Emory University

Part I

Nursing Knowledge and the Challenge of Relevance

Introduction to Part I

Nursing knowledge

Nursing has two faces. To the public, nurses embody the best of modern health care. Efficient, effective, and caring, nurses are at the center of the patient's experience. The other face is largely invisible to the patient, even though it has been a part of nursing since the time of Florence Nightingale. Nursing requires knowledge. In the first century of nursing, the intellectual dimensions of nursing remained implicit. Nurses were trained using an apprenticeship model. Long hours at the bedside were supplemented by some pearls of wisdom dispensed by physicians. By the middle of the twentieth century, it became clear that effective nursing practice required a distinctive body of knowledge. Nursing intervention had gradually become independent of the physician's orders, and nursing required integrated knowledge of the physiological, psychological, and social dimensions of the patient. By developing programs of research, nurses asserted ownership over the knowledge required for practice. Contemporary nursing thus encompasses both the professional practice of nursing and the academic discipline of nursing.

The goal of nursing research is to develop a body of knowledge that will support and advance nursing practice. Nursing knowledge might be defined by its relevance to nurses, an idea suggested by Pamela Reed and Lisa Lawrence:

> *"Nursing knowledge refers to knowledge warranted as useful and significant to nurses and patients in understanding and facilitating human health processes."* (Reed & Lawrence, 2008, p. 423)

While the definition seems clear and straightforward, producing useful and significant knowledge for nurses and their clients has been challenging. The difficulties faced by nurse scholars have gone beyond the ordinary questions of method that concern all researchers. For example, nurse researchers have experimentally demonstrated that one educational intervention promotes adherence to an asthma-monitoring protocol better than another (Burkhart *et al.*, 2007). This is knowledge that is well warranted by its experimental design, and apparently useful to nurses and their patients. However, nurse scholars have not been satisfied by contributions like these. Without deeper links to a growing body of knowledge, such studies have a limited ability to support the intellectual development of nursing. Nor do "qualitative" studies fare any better. Understanding the lived experience of the patient is certainly part of good nursing practice, but without some way of fitting the part into a larger whole, it is difficult to discern the significance of, for example, a description of the lived experience of nine pediatric liver transplant recipients (Wise, 2002). The problem is *not* that studies like these are poorly executed or trivial. On the contrary, they are well designed and important. The problem is that their importance has become difficult to recognize. Working nurses do not seek out the most recent research results or use nursing theories to analyze their responses to the patient. Indeed, the mention of "theory" is likely to elicit groans from a practicing nurse. Nursing theory and research are not supporting the professional practice of nursing in the way that nurses expect it to.

Two kinds of theory–practice gap

The "theory–practice gap" has been discussed in hundreds of nursing articles. This is a symptom of the dissatisfaction nurses seem to have with the research arm of their discipline. But what, exactly, is the theory–practice gap? Historically, the gap has been conceived in two fundamentally different ways. The difference turns on whether existing theory is held to be *relevant* or *irrelevant* to practice. Much writing on the relation of theory to practice assumes that there is a body of relevant intellectual knowledge that should inform nursing practices. The "gap" arises when this body of knowledge is not used as it should be. For example, nursing students often have trouble translating what they learn in the classroom into clinical practice. There is a wealth of literature on pedagogical strategies for helping nursing students bridge this gap. There are other versions of this gap too. Once in professional life, nurses need to continue to learn about new developments, and there are a number of barriers to the integration of research results into nursing practice. The crush of day-to-day work leaves little time for reading and reflection, and there may be no resources to support continuing education. Moreover, theory and research results are not always presented in a form that makes their clinical relevance obvious. These problems are all fundamentally problems of translation. They presuppose that there is a body of useful and relevant knowledge. The theory–practice gap arises when the theory is not translated into action.

The second kind of theory–practice gap is much deeper and more disconcerting. Authors in this vein question the relevance of existing theory and research. For example, in his "Preface" to the fourth edition of *Philosophical and Theoretical Perspectives for Advanced Nursing Practice*, William Cody wrote:

> *"The place of theory in nursing practice has, in reality, long been considered somewhat vague and tenuous. A situation persists today that has been referred to as the*

"theory-practice gap," in which theory and practice are perceived as interacting imperfectly, infrequently, and sometimes insignificantly." (Cody, 2006, p. ix)

In a similar vein, Peter Gallagher[1] wrote:

"[M]any nurses consider it crucial for effective nursing that theory and practice must be closely related. This essentially symbiotic view of the nature of the theory-practice relationship has been embraced by many in the profession, and it is a view that has prompted both expert nurses and inexperienced student nurses to question the direct relevance of some theoretical material to the delivery of nursing care." (Ousey & Gallagher, 2007, p. 200)

These remarks are some of the most recent in a longer tradition (Conant, 1967a, 1967b; Hardy, 1978; Jacobs & Huether, 1978; Watson, 1981; Stafford, 1982; Swanson & Chenitz, 1982; Miller, 1985; Meleis, 1987; Draper, 1990; Nolan & Grant, 1992; Whall, 1993; Good & Moore, 1996; Blegen & Tripp-Reimer, 1997; Im & Meleis, 1999). Unlike those authors who are trying to translate theory into practice, these authors call into question the relevance, significance, or usefulness of existing research and theory. The gap is one of relevance, and this is a disturbing situation. A primary goal—if not the *rasion d'être*—of nursing research is to produce knowledge that supports practice. Since the early 1950s, dozens of journals have published thousands of pages of research reports. If some significant portion of this output supports practice only "imperfectly, infrequently, and sometimes insignificantly," then something is wrong with the research arm of the nursing discipline.

If we follow Reed and Lawrence and define nursing knowledge as knowledge "warranted as useful and significant to nurses" (Reed & Lawrence, 2008, p. 423), then a relevance gap challenges the whole enterprise of nursing research and theory development. If nursing theory were irrelevant, then it would not be nursing knowledge at all. The relevance gap between theory and practice thus raises questions that reach to the foundations of the discipline. It challenges the philosophical conceptions of knowledge that are implicit in the nursing discussions of theory and research. The relevance gap is therefore a fundamental problem of the philosophy of nursing science.

Philosophy of nursing science

The discipline of nursing has a bountiful literature on nursing research, methodology, the character of the nursing discipline, and its substance. These topics are philosophical in the sense that they reflect on the most general and profound issues in nursing scholarship. If we permit ourselves—as we should—a generous understanding of "science," the nursing metatheoretical literature contains substantial work in the philosophy of science. This book aims to contribute to that philosophy

---

[1] While this was a coauthored essay, it was presented as a debate with each author's contribution clearly identified.

of science: to map the intellectual fault lines of nurses' thought about their discipline and to critically engage the issues.

The relevance gap arose at a specific point in the intellectual development of the nursing discipline. As Chapter 1 will show, concern that research or theory might be irrelevant to practice did not arise during the first century of the modern nursing profession. Since the time of Florence Nightingale, nurses have recognized a domain of nursing knowledge, but there was no relevance gap. A relevance gap was recognized by Lucy Conant in the late 1960s (Conant, 1967a, 1967b), but it was not the subject of widespread concern until late 1970s. Why? What caused the gap to open at that point in the history of the discipline? And why has it remained open? Chapter 2 will argue that the relevance gap emerged because of a particular constellation of philosophical ideas. In the 1950s, 1960s, and 1970s, there were debates about the character of nursing knowledge, research, and theory. Toward the end of the 1970s, a consensus about the field emerged. To be a discipline, many thought, nursing needed unique theories at a high level of abstraction. These were unified into a basic science by shared concepts and themes (the metaparadigm). The relevance gap opened because the philosophical understanding of science within nursing urged nurse researchers to develop a basic science, but nursing as basic science had little relevance to the profession.

What is done by philosophy can be undone by philosophy. To close the relevance gap we will have to think through the philosophical arguments about nursing research and theory in which nurse scholars have engaged. This will require attention on two fronts. First, nurse scholars have been influenced by ideas and arguments arising out of philosophy. These will have to be made clear and critically engaged on their own terms. The philosophy of science contains valuable resources for nursing, and several of the chapters below will be devoted to a detailed, critical discussion of issues in the philosophy of science. However, the notions of the philosophers take on a different significance when they enter the nursing context. We cannot restrict ourselves to the philosophers' discussion. The second area of concern will therefore be the nursing literature about the character of the discipline, nursing science, and nursing knowledge. The philosophical position developed here will be intimately related to the debates within nursing. Chapter 3 is intended to be an interface between the philosophy of science and the nursing metatheoretical literature. It will distill four philosophical questions from the nursing debates canvassed in Chapters 1 and 2. It will also sketch, in a preliminary way, the debates to be engaged in this book, and the position that will be developed in subsequent chapters.

Prehistory of the problem

How did the discipline of nursing come to be in a position where significant parts of nursing theory and research are thought to be irrelevant to nursing practice? One might think that the relevance gap arose in the 1970s because only then was there sufficient nursing theory for there to be a theory–practice gap. It would be a mistake to begin the story there. While the development of nursing's research program in the 1950s and 1960s was revolutionary for the profession, theory has been important to nursing since its inception. To understand how the theory–practice gap arose, and why the relevance gap emerged when it did, we have to understand how the relationship evolved between professional nursing and the theories that supported it.

The domain of nursing

Florence Nightingale is praised for her work in identifying the nurse's role in health care, for establishing nurse training, and for her theoretical writing. All three were important for the subsequent development of nursing attitudes toward theory. *Notes on Nursing*: *What It Is and What It Is Not* (Nightingale, [1860] 1969) makes two kinds of contribution to theory. It described a domain of nursing expertise that was independent of the physician's expertise. Specifically, the nurse was oriented toward the environment of the patients, everything from the condition of their bandages to the layout of their sickrooms. From Nightingale forward, then, one kind of theoretical writing in nursing has been to define nursing: to identify the proper scope of the nurse's action, the kinds of nursing response to the patient's needs, and the values that inform nursing actions. Nightingale asked the philosophical question "What is nursing?" and she gave a philosophical answer. She analyzed the nurse's role with an eye toward the values that dictate what it should be (as opposed to the facts about what it is). Nightingale's other theoretical contributions were more empirical. It is often forgotten that in *Notes on Nursing*, Nightingale rejected the germ theory of disease. The germ theory was just emerging in this period, and while it was known as a possible account of disease, it was not widely accepted. Nightingale preferred a late form of the Galenic theory of disease, and she believed that the diseased state of humans sometimes arose directly from their environment (Nightingale, [1860] 1969, pp. 32–34). While this theory of disease did not survive into the twentieth century, it was an important part of Nightingale's justification for the nurse's role. Physicians were to address the problems with the body that caused disease (imbalance of the humors), while nurses addressed the environmental causes. This gave nurses a domain of expertise that fell outside of the physician's domain.

While we can recognize her empirical writings as important theoretical advances in nursing, Nightingale probably would have been reluctant to call them "theory," or to say that nurse training required much in the way of "theory." Indeed, she sometimes expressed a rather ambivalent attitude toward theory. In an 1881 address to the nurses at St. Thomas's Hospital, she wrote:

> *"You are here trained for* nurses—attendants *on the wants of the sick*—helpers *in carrying out doctor's orders (not medical students). Though Theory is very useful when carried out by practice, Theory without practice is ruinous to Nurses."* (Vicinus & Nergaard, 1990, p. 385)

This sentiment was echoed elsewhere in the late nineteenth century nursing literature. In the 1895 essay "Comparative Value of Theory and Practice in Training Nurses," Brennan wrote:

> *"Theory in conjunction with practice is what we want, and although it is undeniable that theory has done more to elevate Nursing than any amount of clinical practice* alone *could have done, we still must remember that 'too much reading tends to mental confusion.'"* (Brennan, 1895, p. 355)

These passages warn nurses against delving too deeply into theory. This is puzzling because both authors clearly think that knowledge of theory is necessary to good nursing. This tension between the need for theory and the danger of too much theory highlights the role that theoretical knowledge played in nineteenth and early twentieth century nursing. Both authors make these remarks while discussing obedience. The role of nurses, both Nightingale and Brennan argued, is to carry out the orders of the physician. The implicit model is that the physicians are the repository of medical and scientific knowledge. To carry out the physician's orders intelligently, nurses must know the medical terminology and enough about medical theories to understand what the physician was asking, and why he was asking for it. The sense in which nurses were enjoined not to read too much, or that theory can be "ruinous," is the sense of "theory" that equates theory with medical knowledge.

Professionalization and the translation gap

The theory required for nursing practice could not be fully identified with medical knowledge, even in Nightingale's time. Nightingale isolated a domain of responsibility where the nurse had expertise. There was, then, a special form of nursing knowledge to be mastered. However, through the late nineteenth and early twentieth centuries, both physicians and nurses expected women to already have this specialized knowledge, at least in part. A young woman with "good upbringing" would already know how to cook and clean, to care for a child or elderly relative, and perhaps to manage domestic help. Her knowledge of the household environment would be refined by apprenticeship in the hospital. The substantive knowledge that was specialized to nursing, contained in works such as *Notes on Nursing: What It Is and Is Not* (Nightingale, [1860] 1969) or *Norris's Nursing Notes: Being a Manual of Medical and Surgical Information for the Use of Hospital Nurses* (Norris, 1891), was largely communicated to the student through experience in the clinic. The knowledge that was specific to nursing was embedded in practice. The pedagogical consequence was that the divide between theory and practice became a divide between knowledge taught in the classroom (or physician's lectures) and knowledge that was acquired in the process of caring for patients. The earliest form of the theory–practice gap, then, was a translation gap. Nurse students and educators faced the challenge of translating medical knowledge into clinical practice.

Throughout the late nineteenth and early twentieth centuries, most of the literature on how theory and practice are related is concerned with pedagogy. Journals for nurses and nurse educators discuss how classroom and clinical work are to be balanced or arranged in the curriculum, and how to test whether the classroom knowledge is being used in the clinical practicum (cf. Norris, 1889, p. 23; McIsaac, 1903; Sellew, 1928). It is a bit surprising, perhaps, that during this period there is *no* literature complaining that theory is irrelevant or useless. Whenever the relation of theory and practice is discussed, the authors presuppose that theory—that is, models of human biology and anatomy, theories about disease etiology, etc.—is relevant to and supports nursing practice. When the theory–practice gap was not strictly pedagogical, it always involved problems of translation. For example, Hyde (1922) complained that what nurses learned in the school setting was often discarded when they entered the profession, not because it was irrelevant, but because the culture of the ward or the pressures of the job kept them from adhering to the ideals they were taught in school. During this period, theory remained relevant to practice partly because nursing stayed in a subservient role. The nurse's job was primarily to carry out the orders of the physician, and knowledge of the physician's theories helped her do so. The relationship between theory and practice was stable for the first hundred years of modern nursing, but its stability was maintained by a relationship of power and authority. The theory–practice relationship changed as the gender dynamics that grounded the physician–nurse relation evolved.

The drive to create a nursing profession was, perhaps, the most important motive for the rise of nursing research. Nursing was not always considered a profession by its practitioners. Nightingale thought of nursing as a vocation, not a profession, and she opposed registration and examination of nurses (Vicinus & Nergaard, 1990, p. 416). In spite of her opposition, nursing organizations pushed for professionalization. The British Nurses Association (established in 1888) and the American Society of Superintendents of Training Schools for Nurses (established in 1893) lobbied for nurses in matters of registration and licensure, educational standards, and working conditions. They initiated the first studies of nursing and established journals for the dissemination of nursing knowledge.

The conception of a profession held by nurses in the first part of the twentieth century was strongly influenced by Dr Abraham Flexner. Flexner was known at the time for his influential study of medical education, and nurse leaders tried (and failed) to get the US Bureau of Education to sponsor a similar study of nursing education (McManus, 1961, p. 77). In 1915, Flexner gave an address at the National Conference of Charities and Correction where he proposed criteria for the status of a profession. A profession, he argued, required "essentially intellectual operations with large individual responsibility" and it must derive its "raw material from science and learning" (Flexner, [1915] 2001, p. 156). Flexner's criteria became the touchstone of nursing discussions about professionalization (cf. Covert, 1917; Roberts, 1925; Bixler & Bixler, 1945; Wolf, 1947, p. 40; Brown, 1948, p. 76). Flexner argued that nursing was not yet a profession (in 1915) because nurses were not sufficiently independent of physicians. "Her function is instrumental," he wrote, "[I]t is the physician who observes, reflects, and decides" (Flexner, [1915] 2001, p. 158). This characterization was disputed by Emily Covert. Covert argued that "nursing is a science" (Covert, 1917, p. 108) with its own literature, that nurse education was moving away from the apprenticeship model, and that the domain of independent nursing responsibility was expanding.

The professional status of nursing was already a topic of lively debate when Flexner made his remarks, so much so that he prefaced them by saying: "I am conscious of endeavoring to pick up a live wire when I undertake to determine the status of the trained nurse" (Flexner, [1915] 2001, p. 158). The dispute about the professional status of nursing involved three related issues: nursing education, the scope of nursing responsibility, and the intellectual basis of nursing. For Flexner and subsequent authors, status as a profession depended on having a domain of independent responsibility. But responsibility alone was insufficient; the responsibility had to have an intellectual basis. Nightingale had already identified the patient's environment as nursing's special responsibility. If nursing was to become a profession, then, the nurse's knowledge of that domain needed to be based on "science and learning" (Flexner, [1915] 2001, p. 156). This meant that nursing education had to move away from hospital-based apprenticeship and into the universities. It also meant that the intellectual basis of nursing action would need to be identified, and ultimately, developed through research.

Nursing education reform in the United States

The main professionalization effort in the first part of the twentieth century was directed toward reform of nursing education. The early nursing schools were affiliated with hospitals. Nurses learned their art primarily through apprenticeship, and hospitals quickly recognized that nursing students provided cheap and plentiful labor. Hospital-affiliated nursing schools thus spread quickly in the English-speaking world. However, the quality of the training varied widely. In the United States, there were many studies of nursing education, of which the Goldmark Report (Committee for the Study of Nursing Education, 1923) and the Brown Report (Brown, 1948) are the most well known. Both were critical of the quality and consistency of nursing schools, and both recommended university-based training for nurses. Brown went so far as to argue for the value of the liberal arts for nurses, in addition to courses in psychology and sociology (Brown, 1948, p. 141).

The move to affiliate nursing schools with universities was an important change. Many nursing schools were very small, and they were staffed by nurses who had been apprenticed, but had no advanced training. Affiliation with universities meant that nurse educators needed advanced degrees. In the 1920s, Teachers College at Columbia University began a masters program in nursing education. Some of these nurses were also trained in research techniques, and they became important contributors to the early study of nursing education (McManus, 1961). There were no doctorates in nursing, and this presented a problem of parity between the faculty of a nursing school and the faculty of the university with which it was affiliated. Brown argued that, if nursing education was to move into the universities, universities would have to permit nurses without PhDs to become professors and directors of nursing programs (Brown, 1948, p. 153). This did not come to pass, and as nursing education became more closely affiliated with colleges and universities, the demand for PhD-trained—and hence, research-trained—nurses increased.

As health care became a more complicated and varied social enterprise, the independence of nurses grew. Public health and private duty nurses had always operated more independently and tended to have more responsibility than their institutional counterparts (Brown, 1948, p. 141). Within hospitals, the medical advances of the early twentieth century made hospital care more elaborate. Nurses were needed to do more than monitor the patient and his or her environment. Nurses were given the responsibility for a variety of actions that were previously restricted to physicians. The domain of nursing activity thus expanded, and nurses were no longer simply carrying out the direct orders of the physician. Nurses were gaining autonomy. At the same time, women were gaining autonomy. World War II saw an influx of women into the workforce in both Great Britain and America. Nursing had helped solidify the notion that women might have a professional life (even if there was a difference between male and female professions). The idea that nursing knowledge could be a simple extension of the woman's household role could no longer be sustained. Nursing required a specialized form of knowledge, and the leaders among nurses recognized that this knowledge needed to be developed through research and taught in a university.

While the need to develop nursing knowledge had been recognized since the early twentieth century, little research was actually carried out. The final push came when the US government began to fund nursing research. During World War II, American government agencies gathered data on the availability and need for nurses. The importance of nurses and their indispensability to modern health care had become widely acknowledged. Because of this recognition, research on nursing became a public funding priority. In 1948, the US Public Health Service created a Division of Nursing Resources, which eventually developed into the National Institute for Nursing Research. Beginning with small grants from the Division of Nursing Resources, funds gradually became available for nursing research. This began a project of research on the education of nurses, on their job satisfaction and turnover, and on nursing functions and activities (McManus, 1961; Gortner, 2000, p. 61). The journal *Nursing Research* was established in 1952, marking the beginning of a full-blown research enterprise.

Nursing research begins

Early nursing research fell, broadly, into three categories. During the early part of the twentieth century, research by and for nurses focused on educational and professional matters. The bulk of the work published in *Nursing Research* during its first decade continued the tradition of examining nurse education, roles, and job responsibilities. This literature was sociologically oriented and was strongly influenced by mid-century trends in sociology. Gradually, however, studies began to appear that either examined the effectiveness of nursing interventions or proposed a useful way of approaching nursing problems. By the early 1960s, this second kind of research had an established place in the literature.

Systematic treatises on nursing were the third kind of nursing research. Hildegard Peplau's *Interpersonal Relations in Nursing* (1952), Ida Jean Orlando's *The Dynamic Nurse–Patient Relationship: Function, Process, and Principles* (1961), Ernestine Wiedenbach's *Clinical Nursing: A Helping Art* (1964), and Virginia Henderson's *The Nature of Nursing* (1966) were among the first of these. These books had several aims. Primarily, they provided an analysis of nurse–patient (and sometimes nurse–family, nurse–nurse, etc.) interactions. They divided the process of nursing into stages and articulated the roles distinctive of nursing. The conceptual framework was intended to facilitate nursing practice and education. Conceptualizing the process was a valuable aid to making explicit nursing problems and their solution. Finally, these works tried to establish what was special, important, or essential to nursing. They aimed to provide the underlying rationale for the existence of the nursing profession.

As the resources and capacity for research grew in the 1940s and 1950s, there was some discussion about the future directions of nursing research. In the first years of its publication, *Nursing Research* ran a regular column asking subscribers about the research topics they thought most important for nursing. The first expression of concern about the kind of research being done in nursing was an editorial by Virginia Henderson in 1956. She pointed out that in the first 4 years of publication, most of the essays in *Nursing Research* had concerned nurses—their education, occupational role, working conditions, etc.—not the science that supported nursing practice (Henderson, 1956). Henderson's generalization was supported by Hortense Hilbert, who surveyed 630 articles published in health journals between 1950 and 1958 (Hilbert, 1959). Henderson and Hilbert were both members of the editorial board for *Nursing Research,* and these leaders were calling for an increase in "clinical nursing research." As they saw it, this research was to be based on the natural and social sciences. Theory was needed too, but this was not yet conceived in the terms that are now familiar to nurses. In their proposal for "An Experimental Program in Nursing Research," Eleanor Sheldon and her colleagues wrote:

> *"Another aspect of nursing research is its lack of theoretical orientation and its strong emphasis on urgency and utilization.... However, if nursing is viewed (as medicine could be viewed also) as a process of assessment and remedial intervention, the nursing research might be conceived of as a sharpening of that assessment perspective, the products from which could yield more efficient and refined remedial intervention—for the ultimate purpose of improving the care of patients. A sharpened perspective in relation to research, however, must be drawn from a theoretical orientation or at least a body of content from which to draw and formulate researchable questions. Members of the nursing profession are not ignorant of the dire necessity for some articulated and systematic fund of knowledge on which to build both its present and future practice."* (Sheldon *et al.*, 1959, pp. 169–170)

It is clear from the content of the proposed program that Sheldon *et al.* were thinking of "theory" as a systematic consolidation of natural and social scientific findings relevant to nursing practice. In the 1950s, then, the call for a new direction in research was a call to move away from educational and occupational research and toward a more systematic investigation into the kinds of theory that had traditionally supported nursing practice.

Nursing research thus developed gradually through the first half of the twentieth century. It arose out of the desire to professionalize nursing, and the belief that a profession needed a unique knowledge base to support independent action in an area of expertise. The existing theories—biological, psychological, and social—were held to be relevant and important for nursing practice. Indeed, Henderson's critique in 1956 was aimed at increasing the engagement of nurses with these established scientific domains, not finding a new frontier for nursing science. Up through the 1950s, there was no concern that nursing research and theory was irrelevant; a relevance gap between theory and practice had yet to arise. This means that the theory–practice gap must be the result of some subsequent development. It also hints that the relevance gap between theory and practice is distinctive of the nursing discipline. It is not a general problem about how academic knowledge is related to practical know-how. If it were, the problem would have arisen during the first hundred years of modern nursing. No, the relevance problem has to do with the way nursing knowledge and the academic discipline of nursing have been conceived, and it is a product of the latter part of the twentieth century.

A philosophy of nursing

The inaugural issue of *Nursing Research* opened with an essay entitled "What is Nursing Research?" (Bixler, 1952). It set the direction for the new journal, articulating a conception of research that was broad and inclusive. Indeed, it was so broad as to call for research in nursing *philosophy*: "There is the greatest dearth at present in the area of philosophical research, in nursing even more than the literature of other professions" (Bixler, 1952). To those of us with a passion for both philosophy and nursing, this allusion is as vexing as it is exciting. Little in the nursing literature before or after Bixler's essay would be recognized by philosophers as a contribution to their field. What could she have meant by "philosophical research?" The clue is provided by the remarks that immediately follow:

> *"Difficult as this kind of [philosophical] research is, it is very necessary and more of it should be produced. In times of rapid social change such as ours, it is dangerous to be charting courses by means of tradition only as a guide. On the basis of directions considered desirable by the leaders of the profession and others, and within the framework of the democratic philosophy as well as known scientific principles, systematic investigation of a projective sort must be undertaken.... It will include schemes for evaluation as well, another aspect of research as yet imperfectly understood and practiced within nursing."* (Bixler, 1952, p. 8)

Bixler's talk of "rapid social change" and the need for direction from "leaders of the profession" indicate that she was referring to the rapidly changing role of nurses. At the beginning of the century, most nurses were employed in private practice. They had responsibility for the complete care of the patient. By the middle of the century, most nurses were employed in hospitals. Nurses had taken over many technical procedures that had been the sole provenance of the physician. More problematically, it also meant that many traditional nursing functions were being handed over to "nonprofessional" staff. Nurses were moving away from direct patient care and into a managerial role (Brown, 1948; Saunders, 1954; Reissman & Roher, 1957). To many nurses, this was a troubling loss. Bixler's call for a philosophy of nursing was thus a call to define nursing, to find its heart, and thereby defend a nurse's proper role.

Concern about the changing role of nurses led a number of mid-century authors to pursue a philosophy of nursing in Bixler's sense. Since it was widely recognized at the time, Bixler was no doubt aware of Sister Olivia Gowan's "definition of nursing":

> *"Nursing in its broadest sense may be defined as an art and a science which involves the whole patient—body, mind, and spirit; promotes his spiritual, mental, and physical health by teaching and by example; stresses health education and health preservation, as well as ministration to the sick; involves the care of the patient's environment—social and spiritual as well as physical; and gives health service to the family and community as well as to the individual."* (Gowan, 1946, p. 10, quotation reprinted in *Nursing Outlook* **7** (4), 199 (1959))

This philosophy of nursing sounded all of the themes on which subsequent definitions would draw (e.g., Henderson, 1966). The other early works that fit Bixler's conception of a philosophy of nursing were the systematic treatises on nursing by Peplau (1952), Orlando (1961), and Wiedenbach (1964). These works helped define nursing by providing an analysis of the nurse's function that was based on an empirical study of nursing activities. Orlando characterized her work in these terms:

> *"The nature of the patient's distress and his need for help are examined in order to identify professional nursing function. The nursing situation is analyzed in terms of its elements (the patient's behavior, the nurse's action and reaction) as they effect the process of helping the patient. From this analysis, principles of effective nursing practice are formulated."* (Orlando, 1961, p. viii)

Orlando expressed the hope that this kind of analysis would contribute to the discussion of "nurse–patient relationships, the nurse's professional role and identity, and the development of knowledge which is distinctly nursing" (Orlando, 1961, p. viii). By the early 1960s, nurse scholars began to think that the relationship between a philosophy of nursing and the development of "distinctly nursing" knowledge was extremely important.[1]

What would a nursing science look like?

The connection between a philosophy of nursing and the larger research enterprise was developed in two influential papers: Dorothy Johnson's "A philosophy of nursing" (1959a) and Rozella Schlotfeld's "Reflections on nursing research" (1960). Both essays voice concerns about the professional role of the nurse. They took the position that nurses ought to be direct caregivers, and they were looking for intellectual grounds on which to resist change to this role. Nursing had been changed, they felt, by "social forces," not by reflective, intentional action by nurses. Since Flexner ([1915] 2001), the intellectual expertise of a profession had been taken to be definitive of its proper domain of action. Both Johnson and Schlotfeld argued that nursing needed to develop its intellectual arm so that the proper role of the nurse could be identified and defended. Up to that point, they felt, the knowledge that supported

---

[1] A charming example is Kathryn Smith's (1960) essay "The new tomorrow in nursing: what the nurse educator sees in her crystal ball." The author gazes into the remote future of 1980. The first thing she sees is: "[T]he nursing profession has met the challenge of its member and allied professions to formulate and to accept a *philosophy of nursing*. With clarity and assurance she can answer the many questions which were asked in 1960: What is nursing? What are appropriate roles for nurses? What are appropriate roles for nursing assistants? How are those roles coordinated to provide integrated patient care of good quality? Are nurses prepared primarily for technical functions? Do nurses do therapy? What is a nursing diagnosis? Where is the bedside nurse? What is the psychotherapeutic function of the nurse?" (Smith, 1960, p. 547, italics in original).

nursing was primarily medical knowledge. In the 1940s and 1950s, nursing education had supplemented the physician's biological knowledge with psychology and sociology. Nursing knowledge had thus grown beyond the boundaries of medical knowledge, but there was, as yet, little that nurses could call their own. Research and theory development were needed to create a knowledge base that would be unique to nursing. By calling for the development of an intellectual domain for nursing and relating it to practice, both Johnson and Schlotfeld were creating the conceptual background for the emergence of a discipline of nursing.

In these essays, Johnson and Schlotfeld also began to articulate the relationship between the discipline of nursing and the professional practice of nursing. They held that nursing research and theory development should be largely autonomous of the practical needs of nurses. The philosophical definition of nursing should set the goal for nursing practice. The knowledge required to achieve those goals would then be the intellectual domain of expertise of the professional nurse. The goals of nursing would thus determine the scope of nursing knowledge and the proper topics for research and theory (Johnson, 1959a, p. 200; Johnson, 1959b, p. 292; Schlotfeld, 1960, p. 493). Nursing research would then develop and test theories about a range of topics, including the health of the patient, the patient's response to nursing intervention, and the nurse–patient interaction. These theories would be the knowledge on which nursing practice would be based. As Sue Donaldson and Dorothy Crowley were to later express the point, "the discipline of nursing should be *governing* clinical practice" (Donaldson & Crowley, 1978, p. 118, emphasis in original).

Johnson and Schlotfeld did not require that nursing theory and research directly respond to the problems of practice. As Myrtle Brown put it, nursing research should aim at "the pursuit of knowledge for the sake of knowledge; its aims should not be limited to the search for facts needed to solve a specific practical problem" (Brown, 1964, p. 111). An alternative view was articulated by a number of scholars, many of whom were associated with the Yale University School of Nursing (e.g., Wald & Leonard, 1964; Conant, 1967a; Dickoff & James, 1968; Ellis, 1969). These authors argued that nursing research needed to be directly responsive to the problems of nursing practice. Some concepts of nursing theory would be drawn from nursing practice. Practicing nurses, Ellis argued, already had substantive knowledge that was relevant to patient care. Nursing research would make some of this knowledge explicit. Established biological, psychological, or social theories would be used to illuminate and expand the practitioner's knowledge. Then nurse researchers would subject the generalizations to clinical test. Since the theory was developed in response to problems recognized by nurses, the knowledge generated by such research would be useful to the nursing profession. Wald and Leonard called this view "practice theory" (Wald & Leonard, 1964). The focus on problem solving, rather than knowledge for knowledge's sake, led to a different conception of the theory–practice relationship. While many writers held that the discipline must govern the practice, practice theorists held that the practice should govern the discipline: "The domain of nursing practice should delimit the domain appropriate to theory development for nursing" (Ellis, 1968, p. 222).

Nursing theory and nursing knowledge

Some nurse scholars worried that a focus on problems in nursing practice would keep nursing research from developing into a proper science. In an essay written for the 10th anniversary of *Nursing Research,* Loretta Heiderken argued that most nursing research up to that point had been "problem-oriented rather than knowledge-oriented" (Heiderken, 1962, p. 141). As a result:

> *"research in nursing is not yet scientific. Problem-solving and research are not synonymous; to be scientific problem-solving in research must proceed from a body of theory (at least a simple conceptual model) and feed back into that theory."* (Heiderken, 1962, p. 141)

This idea that properly scientific research proceeded from and fed back into theory was supported (and perhaps inspired) by mid-century philosophy of science. Beginning in the late 1950s, the nursing literature regularly cited work by philosophers such as Carl Hempel, Hans Reichenbach, Karl Popper, Herbert Feigl, and Ernest Nagel. For these philosophers, the creation and testing of theory was definitive of science. Moreover, scientific theory was supposed to have a particular logical structure: it was a set of abstract and general laws. By specifying values for the variables or other initial conditions, testable hypotheses could be deduced from theory. If the hypotheses conflicted with observation, the theories would have to be modified. Scientific research was thus a matter of theory development and testing. It followed that without theory, nursing research could not be scientific. Brown's essay "Research in the development of nursing theory" (1964) was one of the first works to develop this idea. She argued that nursing researchers needed to clearly show the relationship between their work and some larger theory. Only such a link would unify nursing research projects into a true science of nursing.

Borrowed theory

The perceived need for theories to guide research raised another question: what kind of theory did nurse researchers need? Some were content to draw on existing sciences. Nurse scholars such as Laruie Gunter (1962), Eleanor Sheldon (1963), and Virginia Cleland (1967) held that nursing research should draw on theories from sociology, psychology, physiology, and pathology. Gunter argued that practicing nurses needed sound science on which to base their activities, and some of the knowledge relevant for nursing had already been developed in other disciplines. "These theories alone," Gunter wrote, "will not be unique, but the contribution and the special aspects stressed for each will be unique to nursing in such a manner as to distinguish it (nursing) from other functions" (Gunter, 1962, p. 6). Rosemary Ellis (1968) developed this idea by suggesting that the unique circumstances of nursing would require that these theories be developed and modified. Because the nursing encounter was holistic, theories from different domains would have to be combined. While the theories would be drawn from other disciplines, Gunter (1962, p. 219) and

Sheldon (1963, p. 150) thought that the goals of nursing (as established in a philosophy of nursing) should set the scope of nursing knowledge and determine the selection of relevant theories. In the views of these authors, the disciplinary knowledge required for the profession did not take the form of theories unique to nursing. As Ellis put it, "[W]e strive to act holistically, though our knowledge does not come for use from any holistic science of humans" (Ellis, 1969, p. 1434).

Other nurse scholars rejected the idea that nursing should rely on "borrowed theory." Wald and Leonard (1964, p. 310) argued that, if nursing was to "become an independent 'discipline' in its own right," it would have to free itself from the other sciences and develop its own theory. In her 1968 essay, "Theory in Nursing: Borrowed and Unique," Johnson[2] presented an argument to support the need for a unique nursing theory. The proper boundaries of nursing practice, she argued, need to be established with the cooperation of the wider society, and "society will grant a monopoly of judgment for an area of original responsibility only when there is proof that we have acquired the knowledge needed to solve problems of social significance" (Johnson, 1968, p. 208). The only way to develop such knowledge is through research on the "area of original responsibility." In other words, the unique responsibility of the profession is determined by the unique knowledge base. Therefore, Johnson concluded, the profession of nursing would have secure and sound boundaries only if nursing science could create a distinctive area of intellectual expertise (Johnson, 1968, p. 208).

Uniqueness

If nursing theories are to be unique, then what features distinguish nursing theories from the other sciences? Johnson suggested: "If there is an area for study and theory development unique to nursing, it will evolve only through the study of phenomena and the asking of questions in a way that it not characteristic of any other discipline" (Johnson, 1968, p. 208). Nursing theories are thus distinctive because their content is unique. Johnson's suggestion was important and novel in the nursing literature. The idea that a discipline should have unique subject matter did not get much play in the literature of the 1950s and 1960s. There was general agreement that the subject matter of nursing science should be something about the nursing process, the way that nurses interacted with and influenced the health of their clients. Through the mid-1960s, however, most writers were content to identify the study of nursing process as an "applied science." Wald and Leonard had argued nursing science was not applied (Wald & Leonard, 1964), but they did not propose a unique subject matter for nursing theories. Johnson's essay was thus important because it argued that theories unique to nursing were necessary, and it used the content of nursing theories to identify their uniqueness.

---

[2] In her early work on the character of nursing science, Johnson (1959b, p. 292) was content to think of nursing theory as a "synthesis, reorganization or extension of concepts drawn from the basic and other applied sciences." By 1968, Johnson shared Wald and Leonard's view.

In a series of influential essays, James Dickoff and Patricia James developed Wald and Leonard's idea of a practice theory (Dickoff & James, 1968; Dickoff *et al.*, 1968a, 1968b). Dickoff and James distinguished nursing theory, not by what its theories were about, but what they were *for*. The purpose of nursing theory was to help nurses bring about change. Theories in other disciplines were primarily descriptive and explanatory. Nursing theory needed to build on these other levels of theory, but it must go beyond them insofar as it articulates what makes nursing activity *good*. Nursing theory aimed to identify the goals of nursing practice and show how some kinds of nurse–patient interaction contributed to those goals. The theories specific to nursing science, what Dickoff and James called "situation-producing theory," thus incorporated values. This was a revolutionary suggestion. The common view among scientists and philosophers of science at this time was that science should not include values; science was value-free.[3] Dickoff and James recognized that if a discipline was closely associated with a professional practice (such as nursing, medicine, dentistry, social work, or engineering), it must incorporate some evaluative commitments. Since the purpose of nursing theory was to support the interventions of professional nurses, it required a kind of theory that would articulate the goods of nursing practice. Nursing theory was thus unique not only because it had a distinctive subject matter (the nursing process), but also because it included values.

Conclusion: the relevance gap appears

It was within the intellectual milieu of the late 1960s that a *relevance* gap between theory and practice was first mentioned in the nursing literature. In two essays (Conant, 1967a, 1967b), Lucy Conant expressed the concern that nursing theory and research were not sufficiently useful to the practitioner:

"Research frequently is seen as being a desirable activity in itself, regardless of its purpose and nature. The result of this thinking is that nursing research is not necessarily evaluated in terms of its contribution to nursing practice. At the same time there are many problems in practice that are being ignored by nurse researchers because of their distance from the realities and complexities of nursing. The result is that there is a wide gap between the nurse researcher and the nurse practitioner, as neither sees the other as having a useful contribution to make to her own interests and concerns. If this separation should continue, it could lead ultimately to the deterioration of both nursing practice and nursing research." (Conant, 1967b, p. 114)

For the first time, the concern about the relationship of theory and practice is not a matter of either pedagogy or of translating scientific discoveries into useful bedside practices. Rather, researchers are said to be "ignoring" the needs of practitioners,

---

[3] It should be pointed out, however, that this view had been already challenged and there was debate about it within the philosophy of science (Rudner, 1953; Churchman, 1956; Jeffery, 1956; Levi, 1960). These arguments will be discussed in Chapter 5.

and professional nurses are said to think that nursing research and theory are useless. Conant made these points in the course of arguing against the "knowledge for knowledge's sake" perspective on nursing theory and research. On the contrary, she was arguing, theory needed to be in the service of practice, and should be evaluated by its contribution to practice. Like Dickoff and James, she thought that nursing theory incorporated values: "Scientific theory is descriptive and predictive, while practice theory must not only describe and predict but also prescribe the activities of the practitioner" (Conant, 1967b, p. 114). Conant's articulation of the relevance gap between theory and practice was thus part of an argument that *unless* nursing theory and research were conceptualized along the lines of practice theory, nursing theory was doomed to be irrelevant.

While Conant's presentation of the relevance gap is clear, the idea lay dormant in the nursing literature for 10 years. Conant's essays were critically discussed, but subsequent nurse scholars did not reaffirm her expression of the gap. It was 1978 before Margret Hardy would complain that "grand theories" provide "no practical foundation for nursing practice" (Hardy, 1978, p. 42), and it was the 1980s before concern about the theory–practice gap became widespread. Conant's presentation of the relevance gap, then, was like Henderson's question: "Research in Nursing Practice—When?" (Henderson, 1956). Both were ahead of their time in sensing that there was something wrong with the direction of nursing research. The stage was set, but the play would have to unfold before the audience would discover what, exactly, was rotten in Denmark.

Opening the relevance gap

In the 1970s, nurse scholars made a philosophical choice. They chose to adopt a particular philosophical understanding of science. A consensus grew about the character of nursing theory and research, nursing knowledge, and the relationship between the discipline of nursing and the professional practice of nursing. That consensus remains pervasive and influential today, framing the debate about the character of nursing knowledge. It could have been otherwise; there was another conception of nursing science available in the late 1960s. What would nursing science look like in the light of a different philosophy of science? Can the road not taken be recovered and reconstructed?

Two conceptions of nursing science

In the 1960s, the movement to create a nursing research discipline raised three interrelated issues: (1) the relationship of nursing theory and research to practice, (2) whether the discipline of nursing required unique theories, and if so, (3) what the special character of nursing theories might be. In the early 1970s, opinions about these issues had coalesced into two camps.

On one side were those who defended some form of "practice theory." The name was first used by Wald and Leonard (1964), and discussions of practice theory usually mentioned work by Ellis (1968, 1969), Conant (1967a, 1967b), Dickoff and James (1968), and Dickoff *et al.* (1968a, 1968b). These authors held that nursing research and theory should be directly responsive to the needs of professional practice. Nurses and nurse administrators should determine the appropriate scope and character of professional practice. The role of the discipline was to provide the knowledge needed by the practice. While the practice theorists rejected the idea that nursing was an applied science, they were tolerant of borrowed theory. To address the problems of professional nursing, research would draw on the existing sciences, especially biology, sociology, and psychology.

Practice theorists identified the distinctive character of nursing knowledge in two ways. First, nursing problems were complex; they required the integration of knowledge about the biological, psychological, and social aspects of the person or nurse–client interaction. So, a theory derived from one discipline would have to be integrated into theories from other disciplines, and this would create knowledge distinctive of nursing. Second, nursing theory had to prescribe, not just describe. The aim of theory and research was to guide practice, so theory development had to incorporate nursing values. Dickoff and James argued that nurse scholars could not simply accept the goals of the profession. Nursing values and goals required criticism and testing, and this required knowledge of the causal systems with which nursing practice engaged. Therefore, development of nursing goals and values was an integral part of theory development.

Practice theory was roundly criticized in the 1970s. Out of the criticism, a consensus grew around a different conception of nursing knowledge. On this view, nursing is a basic science. Nursing theory is unique because it studies a distinctive set of topics. Like physics, sociology, or biology, the discipline of nursing was to be defined by its subject matter. The knowledge developed by the discipline is the intellectual expertise that defines the nursing profession. In this way, the discipline was to govern the professional practice of nursing. Through the 1970s and into the early 1980s, a number of theories were developed that were intended to be general theories of nursing: Betty Newman (1982), Martha Rogers (1970), Margaret Newman (1986), Imogene King (1971), Sister Calista Roy (1976), and Rosemarie Rizzo Parse (1981). The work of earlier authors, such as Wiedenbach (1964), Orlando (1961), and Peplau (1952), was interpreted[1] as having a similar aim. By the late 1970s, practice theory was no longer a viable way of conceptualizing nursing knowledge. The future direction of the nursing discipline was to propose general theories about the distinctive topics of nursing (grand theory), and then develop more concrete theories that would support nursing interventions (middle-range theory).

Chapter 1 argued that nurses did not recognize a relevance gap between theory and practice prior to Conant's 1967 essay "Closing the practice–theory gap." Even after Conant's essay defined the gap, it was another decade before the gap was widely recognized as a problem. This means that the relevance gap opened just as nurse scholars were settling on the idea that nursing is a basic science, and fixing their ideas about the character of nursing knowledge, research, and theory. Is there a relationship between the philosophical ideas that developed in the 1970s and the perception of a relevance gap? To answer this question, we need to look a bit more closely at the arguments that brought down practice theory and solidified the idea that nursing is a basic science.

---

[1] It will be argued in Chapter 15 that this interpretation misrepresented the early theorists in important ways.

The demise of practice theory

In 1971, Lorraine Walker published "Toward a clearer understanding of the concept of nursing theory" in *Nursing Research* (Walker, 1971). The essay was a broad critique of earlier nursing conceptions of scientific theory, including practice theory. The character of theory was a hot issue; Folta described the atmosphere among nurse theorists at the time as "electrifying" (Folta, 1997). Lucile Notter, editor of *Nursing Research*, took the unprecedented step of inviting responses to Walker prior to the publication of her essay. The essay presented two key philosophical ideas: scientific theory is value-free, and scientific theories have a distinctive logical structure. Both of these ideas were well entrenched in mid-century philosophy of science, and they were developed in the nursing literature throughout the 1970s.

The argument from value freedom

Walker's essay began by drawing a firm distinction between the "description and explanation of what occurs in a given state-of-affairs" and the identification of "worthy means and ends for a given practical endeavor" (Walker, 1971, p. 428). The former is "scientific" theory, the latter "philosophical." Questions about what forms of nursing practice are effective can be answered by settling on the goals of nursing (a philosophical question) and then empirically determining the most effective way of achieving those ends (a scientific question). Calling questions about effective nursing practice "praxiology," Walker remarked:

> "It is important to note that though, for instance, science of nursing may facilitate the development of praxiology of nursing, each of these three modes of discourse [science, philosophy, and praxiology] represent essentially non-integrated or independent theories of nursing." (Walker, 1971, p. 429)

Walker thus separated questions of fact from questions of value, assigning each to an independent realm of discourse. This conclusion directly opposed the main idea of practice theory. The practice theorists had argued that nursing theories needed to develop principles of practice, and to do so, nursing theory would have to integrate the values of practice with the science. Walker's division of science, philosophy, and praxiology was thus at odds with practice theory.

In their response to Walker, Dickoff and James pointed out that Walker's argument relied on special definitions of "science," "praxiology," and "philosophy," and that these definitions were adopted without argument (Dickoff & James, 1971). If Walker's definitions are used, then "practice theory" becomes a misnomer; but why accept Walker's stipulations? Practice theorists had already defended a different way of thinking about science, philosophy, and praxiology. Walker's separation of science from the study of nursing values needed argumentative support.

Jan Beckstrand provided arguments supporting Walker in a series of philosophically informed essays (Beckstrand, 1978a, 1978b, 1980). Her main argument was that there were two possible roles for values in practice theory: (1) as an ethics for the profession or (2) as goals for the practice. Empirical science is irrelevant to an ethics for the profession, she argued. No amount of empirical research into what *is* the case will tell us how things *ought* to be. Hence, the values of the profession are subject to philosophical discussion, not scientific research. The question of goals may be divided into two elements: the goals to be obtained, and the means for obtaining them. Again, choice of goals is a strictly evaluative matter to which science has little to contribute. However, once the goals were established, scientific inquiry could determine the best way to achieve them. According to Beckstrand, then, practice theory could only be praxiology: the instrumental use of science to achieve the goals of the profession.

The argument from theory structure

Practice theorists had contended that nursing practice was an important resource for nursing theory. Ellis pointed out that practitioners already had knowledge of how to effectively nurse. On her view, nursing theory should make this knowledge explicit (Ellis, 1969). Conant thought that research needed to respond to nursing problems and that theory should provide practical direction for nurses (Conant, 1967b). Walker argued that this sort of work did not really constitute scientific theory:

> "A theory may be differentiated from other forms of knowledge by, among other things: (1) the nature of the terms used, and (2) the character of its internal relations. The terms within a theory are 'systematically related,' that is, logically related, such that deductions from certain fundamental statements to other derived statements become possible. The nature of the terms within the theory are general, and thus form an organizational scheme for describing and explaining certain recurrent existential state-of-affairs." (Walker, 1971, p. 432)

Walker here expresses a view about theory that was prevalent in the 1950s and 1960s. In the technical jargon of the time, this was a "deductive–nomological" conception of theory. (Later, it came to be called "the received view of theory.") According to this view, scientific theory was a body of natural laws. The laws might be expressed as universal generalizations (e.g., for every action, there is an equal and opposite reaction) or mathematical formulas (e.g., $F = ma$). From these laws, more restricted generalizations could be deduced using mathematics and logic. Theories thus form a hierarchy, with the most abstract and general theories at the top, and less general, more concrete theories below. To mid-century philosophers of science, the goal of science was to produce and test theory, and all properly scientific theorizing had this deductive–nomological form.

Walker was not the only nurse theorist to be attracted to a deductive–nomological conception of theory. By the early 1970s, it was widespread among nurse scholars. Works by Faye Abdellah (1967), Imogene King (1971), Marjorie Batey (1971), Margret Newman (1972), Ada Jacox (1974), Joan Riehl and Sister Callista Roy (1974), and Dorothy Johnson (1974) developed this conception of theory and applied it to nursing.[2] The deductive–nomological conception of theory had important consequences for the relation of theory to practice. On the deductive–nomological view, concrete and specific regularities were predicted by deducing them from more abstract laws. Jacox (1974) argued that the principles that support nursing practice should be narrow generalizations deduced from more general theory. As an example, she used the generalization that a lack of oxygen causes tissue breakdown. This is a proposition of biological theory. It is general in the sense that it is true of a large class of biological organisms. From this theoretical proposition, along with other definitions and propositions of the theory, it follows that if prolonged decreased circulation to a part occurs, a decubitus ulcer will form. This describes a specific relationship between a human health problem (decubitus ulcer) and its cause. Knowing the specific principle, and given the goal of enhancing human health, a practicing nurse knows how to act (Jacox, 1974).

As a result of these two arguments—that nursing science and nursing values are independent, and that properly scientific theories have a deductive–nomological structure—practice theory was gradually eclipsed in the nursing literature during the 1970s. Proponents of practice theory did respond (Dickoff & James, 1971; Ellis, 1971; Collins & Fielder, 1981), but the weight of opinion, at least as expressed in the literature, was against them. A consensus began to coalesce around the idea that nursing is a basic science.

The consensus emerges

In 1978, three essays were published that crystallized the conception of nursing as a basic science: Barbara Carper's "Fundamental patterns of knowing in nursing," Sue Donaldson and Dorothy Crowley's "The discipline of nursing," and Jacqueline Fawcett's "The relationship between theory and research: a double helix." This body of work became the reference point for later discussion of nursing theory and research.

Carper's patterns of knowledge

Carper's essay analyzed the kinds of knowledge required by practicing nurses, and used this analysis to show how the knowledge base of the nursing discipline should be organized. She divided nursing knowledge into "empirics," "ethics," "esthetics" (aesthetics), and "personal knowledge" (Carper, 1978). This classification of nursing knowledge had several important consequences. First, it clearly separated ethical knowledge from empirical knowledge. Empirics, according to Carper, was the domain of scientific knowledge: "knowledge about the empirical world, knowledge that is systematically organized in to general laws and theories for the purpose of

---

2 Even Dickoff and James (1968) employ this conception of theory. The difference between their view and the other theorists cited here is that they regarded value-laden "situation-producing theory" as a higher level of theory, built upon the results of deductive–nomological theories.

describing, explaining and predicting phenomena of special concern to the discipline of nursing" (Carper, 1978, p. 14). Ethics, on the other hand, is "focused on matters of obligation or what ought to be done" (Carper, 1978, p. 20). Like Walker and Beckstrand, Carper held that ethical knowledge and scientific knowledge were independent. Value judgments are not amenable to scientific inquiry; scientific inquiry should not be influenced by values.

The second important consequence of Carper's analysis was that it drew a strong distinction between empirical knowledge and practical knowledge. The categories of aesthetics and personal knowledge are both kinds of practical knowledge, of "knowing how" rather than "knowing that." The key elements of the aesthetic component in nursing are that it is particular, rather than general, that it is holistic in the sense of understanding particulars in relation to each other, that it involves empathy, and that it resists discursive formulation. Finally, personal knowledge is a kind of self-awareness that concerns the relationship of self to other. These features distinguish aesthetics and practical knowledge from the law-like generalizations of empirics. Nursing science, as Carper conceives of it, could not directly address issues of practice because these involve forms of knowledge that are not discursive or generalizing.

Donaldson and Crowley on the discipline

While Carper's essay focused on the structure of nursing knowledge, Donaldson and Crowley turned to the structure of a discipline. They contended that there are two kinds of discipline: "academic" and "professional" (Donaldson and Crowley, 1978, p. 115). Professional disciplines support a related profession, such as law, medicine, social work, or nursing. Professional disciplines cannot, therefore, limit themselves to disinterested description of phenomena. They must prescribe. This means that the professional disciplines have a value orientation that the academic disciplines lack. Donaldson and Crowley did not follow the practice theorists in recommending a special kind of value-laden theory for nursing. Rather, the social relevance and value orientation of the discipline is shared with the profession. This value orientation determines the distinctive perspective of the discipline (Donaldson & Crowley, 1978, p. 118). Within this value orientation, the empirical science of nursing can develop. They suggested that the discipline of nursing was unified by interest in three themes (Donaldson & Crowley, 1978, p. 113):

1. Concern with the principles and laws that govern the life processes, well-being, and optimum functioning of human beings—sick or well.
2. Concern with the patterning of human behavior in interaction with the environment in critical life situations.
3. Concern with the processes by which positive changes in health status are affected.

The discipline of nursing was thus aligned with other disciplines in the academy. Any discipline, they argued, was a body of knowledge oriented toward particular interests and framed by a related set of concepts. Inquiry into the subject matter proceeds scientifically, and like any other science, it may take "basic" and "applied" forms. In this way, Donaldson and Crowley were able to identify "the essence of nursing research and of the common elements and threads that give coherence to an identifiable body of knowledge" (Donaldson & Crowley, 1978, p. 113).

While practice helped give the discipline its unique perspective, it did not define its limits, according to Donaldson and Crowley. The discipline of nursing and the professional practice of nursing remained independent. Donaldson and Crowley gave several arguments to support the idea that "the discipline of nursing should be *governing* clinical practice rather than being defined by it" (Donaldson & Crowley, 1978, p. 118, italics in original). First, by 1978, there were nurses writing on nursing history, nursing ethics, and nursing philosophy, in addition to the more practical matters of client interventions and nurse management. The discipline thus had a scope that was broader than the profession. Moreover, as Carper emphasized, nursing practice requires attention to the particular client. But the competencies required for clinical practice draw on a broad understanding of health. Therefore, the discipline needs to direct practice, not *vice versa*. Donaldson and Crowley thus crystallized an idea that had been evolving in the nursing literature for 20 years: the discipline of nursing was a basic science that, when applied to problems of practical nursing, could yield specific direction.

Fawcett on the levels of theory

Fawcett's contribution to the consensus was to create a map of the discipline out of the 1970s view of theory. According to many nurse scholars of the time, scientific theories were sets of propositions or law-like generalizations. They may be more or less abstract, and at their most abstract, Fawcett gave them the status of "conceptual models" (Fawcett, 1980a). All theory must be testable by observations, and to test a very abstract theory, the concepts must be made more concrete and specific. Ultimately, hypotheses are derived that contain operationally defined terms, and these can be tested by observation or experiment (Fawcett, 1978). Fawcett emphasized the idea that research counts as scientific only insofar as it aims at the development or testing of theory. Because all theory fits into a hierarchy—with conceptual models as the most abstract, followed by mid-range theory, then application—all proper scientific research in nursing must be linked to a nursing theory. Fawcett followed Donaldson and Crowley in identifying nursing theories as those that engage a particular set of topics. Indeed, she refined Donaldson and Crowley's three themes by highlighting four concepts woven through them: person, environment, health, and nursing (Fawcett, 1984, p. 84). These four concepts and three themes constituted the "metaparadigm" of nursing, that is, they were the phenomena to be studied by any research and theory that was rightly considered part of the nursing discipline.

Fawcett's essays in the late 1970s and early 1980s provided a philosophical understanding of earlier "grand theory," and made it an integral, necessary part of nursing science (Fawcett, 1980a, 1980b, 1984). While the first systematic treatises on nursing were oriented toward an analysis of the nursing process and nurse–client relationships, nursing theory of the 1970s and 1980s had become removed from the details of nursing practice. Rogers (1970), for example, proposed a holistic "theory of man" that used "principles of homeodynamics" as its main theoretical postulates. Rogers's student, Margret Newman, proposed a theory of health as "expanding consciousness" (Newman, 1986). Systems theory, a very abstract and general theory developed in the social sciences, was brought into nursing by Betty Newman (1982), Imogene King (1971), and Sister Callista Roy (1976). This work was not intended to provide useful information for nurses at the bedside. On the understanding of nursing theory that coalesced during the 1970s, this distance from practice was no vice. Indeed, it was a virtue: basic science should not be expected to provide practical direction. These works were the grand theories or conceptual models that provided nursing science with its most general laws and concepts. This view of theory was captured by the 1980s textbooks on nursing theory, and it continues to be affirmed in recent editions (Chinn & Kramer, [1983] 1999; Walker & Avant, [1983] 2005; Fawcett, [1985] 1999; Meleis, [1985] 2007).

The relevance gap

The relevance gap between theory and practice appeared because of a philosophical view of nursing knowledge. According to the consensus, the basic science of nursing grounds professional practice. The topics and concepts of the metaparadigm determine the unique perspective of the discipline. Within this metaparadigm, conceptual models or grand theories provide the most abstract generalizations. Middle-range theories are either "creatively invented within the hermeneutic context of the theory or logically deduced from the existing structure" (Cody, 1999, p. 11). Applications were supposed to be derived from middle-range theory. This philosophical view took grand theory to be the highest form of nursing science. Nurse scholars were encouraged to formulate their theories in terms distant from the contingencies of practice. There was no need to work directly with clinical concerns. Theory came first; application was left for the future. As a result, nurses at the bedside saw theory and research drift farther and farther away from clinically accessible anchor points.

The new theories of nursing did not satisfy all nurse scholars. While grand theory was being validated as the basic science of nursing, some nurses expressed concern about the new direction. In Hardy's discussion of the nursing theory, she commented that grand theories "provide neither solid nor practical foundations for nursing practice" (Hardy, 1978, p. 42). Stafford wrote that as a clinician she found the unitary man framework "ineffective, cumbersome and time consuming · · · A futile exercise in words and an exercise lacking in specificity" (Stafford, 1982, p. 268). British nurses and nurse scholars seemed particularly puzzled by a kind of theorizing that they took to be an American phenomenon (Miller, 1985; Draper, 1990). In a comprehensive discussion, Audrey Miller identified a number of barriers that kept practicing nurses from appreciating and applying nursing theory (Miller, 1985). These included not only the obscurity of the theorists' language, but also more substantial barriers. She argued that theorists overemphasized general principles and views about how nursing ought to be. Practicing nurses needed interventions and concrete background knowledge that would help care for patients. Theory, some argued, was simply not supplying the knowledge nurses required (Watson, 1981; Stafford, 1982; Swanson & Chenitz, 1982; Miller, 1985; Meleis, 1987; Draper, 1990). Foreshadowed by Lucy Conant in 1967, a relevance gap between nursing theory and nursing practice was clearly recognized in the 1980s.

The qualitative research movement

For a discipline so closely related to practice, a relevance gap is a significant problem. Those who recognized the gap sought ways to close it. One of the early diagnoses of the gap pointed at the philosophical views about science that underlay theory development in the 1970s. Jean Watson remarked that:

> *"Nursing seems to be suffering in its quest for a scientific foundation for its practice. Like the mythological Danaids who kept filling their jars with water only to have it leak through the holes, nursing finds its search for scientific underpinnings as elusive as the liquid."* (Watson, 1981, p. 413).

Watson suggested that nursing had failed to find "scientific underpinnings" for practice because research and theory development had modeled itself after the natural sciences. Janice Swanson and Carole Chenitz, reiterated this idea, contending that "Quantitative nursing research does not have meaning for the practice world of nursing" (Swanson & Chenitz, 1982, p. 241). These nursing scholars sought an alternative kind of nursing research and theory: qualitative theory, not quantitative.

The idea that qualitative research was especially suited to the nursing discipline was given a boost by Patricia Benner's very popular book, *From Novice to Expert* (1984). Carper had already distinguished science (empirics) as a pattern of knowledge different from aesthetics and personal knowledge. The latter were forms of knowledge embedded in practice, and Benner's work argued that the goal of nursing research and theory should be to make explicit the knowledge that is embedded in practice. A number of essays followed, arguing that since "knowing how" and "knowing that" were different forms of knowledge, and nursing practice was a form of know-how, nursing research had to take a new direction (Clarke, 1986; Lauder, 1994; Allmark, 1995; Carr, 1996; Johnson & Ratner, 1997; Penney & Warelow, 1999; Ousey & Gallagher, 2007).

One of the motivations behind qualitative research, then, was to close the relevance gap. Proponents of qualitative research in the 1980s often criticized the philosophical consensus of the 1970s. They argued that theories did not always have a deductive–nomological structure, that observation was influenced by theory, and that values were integral to scientific research. Qualitative research, they argued, developed holistic theories and was value-laden. The proponents of qualitative research, then, were criticizing exactly the philosophical presuppositions that had led to the relevance gap. The debate between qualitative and quantitative researchers was lively in the 1980s. In spite of the criticism, however, the philosophical presuppositions remained in place; the idea that nursing was a basic science did not disappear. Rather, the criticisms were taken to show that qualitative and quantitative research had different philosophical foundations. This led to a rapprochement between qualitative and quantitative researchers. Since both kinds of research could be used to study the themes and topics of the metaparadigm, both contributed to nursing knowledge. However, because of the differences between qualitative and quantitative research, many argued that the two could not be mixed. A debate over "mixed methods" research simmered through the 1980s and 1990s. What began as a radical critique ended up assimilated into the mainstream.

The middle-range theory movement

The qualitative research movement was not the only response to the relevance gap. In the 1990s, proponents of middle-range theory also argued that the consensus view had led to a relevance gap. Nurse scholars inherited the phrase "middle-range theory" from Robert Merton (1957). He had intended it to fit the deductive–nomological picture. Middle-range theories specified the abstract concepts of grand theory, and they formulated more specific, causal hypotheses. The theory literature of the 1970s used the phrase in this way (Walker, 1971; Jacox, 1974; Fawcett, 1978). In the 1990s, middle-range theory took off as a methodological movement in nursing. Dozens of essays promoted middle-range theory, and it was very common for the essays to begin by bemoaning the relevance gap. The opening passage of Marion Good and Shirley Moore's "Clinical practice guidelines as a new source of middle-range theory" was typical:

> "Despite 30 years of concerted effort to develop theory in nursing, there are few theories to support research-based practice by nurses. For example, there are many broad conceptual models of nursing, but no prescriptive nursing theories of pain management. If nursing is to expand its development as a scientific discipline, there is a priority to create middle-range theories from which testable hypotheses can be developed." (Good & Moore, 1996, p. 74)

Development of middle-range theory was the new blueprint for closing the theory–practice gap.

The 1990s enthusiasm for middle-range theory was infused with some important philosophical work. One of the most cited essays about middle-range theory is "Collaborative development of middle-range theories: toward a theory of unpleasant symptoms" by Elizabeth Lenz and her colleagues (Lenz *et al.*, 1995). The second author of this essay was Frederick Suppe, a prominent philosopher of science. Suppe had been a critic of the philosophy of science that had informed the nursing literature during the 1960s and 1970s. His edited volume, *The Structure of Scientific Theories* (Suppe, 1974), documented the arguments against the deductive–nomological conception of scientific theory and related ideas of "the received view." In the 1980s, he was one of a number of philosophers who were developing alternative conceptions of scientific theory (Suppe, 1989). Suppe was an active collaborator with nurse scholars, and he wrote or cowrote several essays that were critical of grand theory and the basic science conception of nursing (Suppe &

Jacox, 1985; Jacox & Suppe, 1990; Suppe, 1993; Lenz *et al.*, 1995, 1997). Suppe's background highlights an often-overlooked feature of the famous "Theory of Unpleasant Symptoms" essay: it *rejects* Merton's conception of middle-range theory. The authors articulate a conception of theory different from the deductive–nomological model (Lenz *et al.*, 1995, p. 3). In their conception, middle-range theory does not make grand theory more concrete. Middle-range theory development was to replace the whole enterprise of developing grand theories (or conceptual models).[3]

While "middle-range theory" became the buzzword of the 1990s, the philosophical critique on which it was based was eclipsed. Middle-range theories tended to draw on the intellectual resources of other disciplines, and this raised concerns about the distinctiveness of the nursing discipline. If the nursing discipline became a hodgepodge of middle-range theories, there would be no unity to the knowledge, no area of intellectual expertise that nurses could call their own. Nurse scholars thus argued that if nursing was to develop as a science, middle-range theories had to be fit within the context of grand theories or conceptual models (Fawcett, [1985] 1999; Cody, 1999). In spite of the intentions of some of the original proponents, then, middle-range theory came to be understood in traditional, Mertonian terms as a kind of theory midway between the abstractions of grand theory and the needs of nursing practice (Phillips, 1996; Liehr & Smith, 1999; Higgins & Moore, 2000; Fawcett, 2005b; Parse, 2005). Recent textbook presentations (Smith & Liehr, 2003; Peterson & Bredow, 2008) have continued to treat middle-range theory in this way. Like qualitative research, then, the middle-range theory movement began as a revolution that criticized the prevailing philosophy of science in nursing. Like so many revolutions, it ended up just as another part of the *status quo*.

Conclusion: the relevance gap endures

There were two major attempts to close the relevance gap: the qualitative research movement and the middle-range theory movement. It is important to note that both began with a deep philosophical criticism of the prevailing view. This shows that nurse scholars in the 1980s and 1990s recognized that the relevance gap had philosophical roots. In the end, as we have seen, neither was able to reverse the trend. Both were assimilated to the existing philosophical framework.

The relevance gap remains as strong as ever, and concern with the gap in the nursing literature shows no sign of abating (Rolfe, 1998; Upton, 1999; Warms & Schroeder, 1999; Larsen *et al.*, 2002; Schwartz-Barcott *et al.*, 2002; Stevenson, 2005; Doane & Varcoe, 2005; Gardner, 2006; Litchfield & Jónsdóttir, 2008). It has become such an established part of the intellectual landscape that some see it as inevitable (Larsen *et al.*, 2002; Ousey & Gallagher, 2007), or even in some respects desirable

---

[3] In Chapter 13, we will consider the character of middle-range theory in more detail.

(Cody, 1999). The Editor-in-Chief of *The American Journal of Nursing*, the oldest nursing journal in America, opened a recent editorial with these remarks:

> *"Say 'nursing science' to many nurses and they'll roll their eyes, remembering the seemingly useless theory and research courses they've sat through. And it's true: Theory and research have too often been irrelevant to the daily practice of nurses."* (Mason, 1999, p. 7)

Mason goes on to argue that current research has much value for practice, but the remark and its placement are striking. We have come a long way from the optimism of the 1950s and 1960s. If the first editorial boards of *Nursing Research* had come to the conclusion that theory and research were irrelevant to the daily practice of nurses, they would have regarded their journal as a failure. It is a tragedy that a profession as important as nursing should struggle to link scientific knowledge to its domain of professional responsibility.

There is some hope. Nursing has a relevance gap between theory and practice because of the philosophical choices made by nurse scholars. The dominant understanding of nursing science is a framework of philosophical theses about science. None of these theses are necessary; all have viable alternatives in the philosophy of science. Indeed, we have seen how some philosophical alternatives were recognized and put forward at crucial junctures in the history of nursing research and theory. And since the 1970s, the philosophy of science has developed and strengthened alternative ways of thinking about science. The relevance gap between theory and practice has opened because of philosophy. Therefore, to close the gap, we need to engage the philosophy of science that is embedded in the nursing literature. We need to build a systematic, philosophical understanding of nursing science that will provide a new perspective on the intellectual foundations of the nursing profession.

Toward a philosophy of nursing science

Nursing inquiry has been shaped by philosophy. At crucial points in the history of nursing research, nurse scholars raised philosophical questions, and their answers shaped the discipline. Chapters 1 and 2 argued that the relevance gap between theory and practice arose because of ideas about how science ought to proceed. The historical discussion also suggested that mid-century philosophy of science influenced nurse scholars in specific ways. Philosophical ideas about science have evolved substantially since the 1970s. Therefore, an important part of rethinking the relationship between the discipline of nursing and the professional practice of nursing—and thus truly addressing the relevance gap—will be to bring recent philosophical views to bear on the nursing literature.

To some extent, new philosophical thinking has been done in nursing under the labels of "postpositivism," "pragmatism," "feminism," and "critical theory." To fully develop an alternative to the current consensus, however, we need to go beyond the isms. The issues cannot be resolved by adopting one or another off-the-rack philosophical view. The idea that a philosophical position can be taken up or discarded like a suit of clothes has stunted too much philosophical work in nursing. Nursing philosophy has to be developed from within nursing. This means using the resources of the philosophy of science to address the questions that have arisen for nurses, and responding to the concerns that have motivated nurse scholars' answers to them. The writings of philosophers of all stripes, from Heidegger to Kuhn, Dewey to Harding, are useful just insofar as they help us articulate and critically defend answers to the fundamental questions of nursing philosophy. We do not need another ism, we need answers.

Philosophical questions about nursing

Questions about the discipline

To imagine an alternative philosophy of science for nursing is to imagine different answers to the philosophical questions that have framed the discipline. The first step, then, must be to uncover the questions. The most prominent philosophical question about nursing research and theory has been:

1. How is the knowledge developed in the discipline of nursing related to the professional practice of nursing?

The twentieth century expansion of nursing research was driven by nurses' desire to create an intellectual basis for their profession. Disciplinary knowledge did more than merely inform practice: the legitimacy of nursing as an autonomous profession depended on having an independent knowledge base. Health care changed substantially in the twentieth century, and this put pressure on the nursing roles. As we saw in Chapter 1, nurses looked to research to help articulate the proper bounds of practice. However, if the distinctive domain of nursing practice is to be set by nursing knowledge, then the knowledge base must be unique. This raises another philosophical question:

2. What is nursing's unique area of intellectual expertise?

In other words, what makes the nursing discipline distinctive? What is the special contribution of the nurse to a research group or health care team? What makes the knowledge deployed by nurses *nursing* knowledge?

We saw in Chapter 2 how different answers to this pair of questions led to a debate among nursing scholars during the 1960s and 1970s. On one side were the practice theorists. They argued that the discipline needed to be closely tied to nursing practice in two ways. First, the problems of nursing research need to be derived from nursing practice. Second, because practical problems presuppose goals and values, these needed to be part of nursing inquiry. The practice theorists thus answered question (1) by making theory directly responsive to the needs of practice. The practice theorists had a bit more trouble with question (2). On their view, the unique character of nursing knowledge is (in part) that it articulates what good nursing amounts to. However, because other disciplines helped address nursing problems, borrowed theories were relevant parts of nursing knowledge. This made it more difficult to explain why nursing was a distinct science. And that problem, in turn, made it difficult to use disciplinary knowledge to determine the proper boundaries of the nursing roles.

The other side of the debate answered question (2) by taking nursing to be a basic science. Like other basic sciences, it had a unique domain set by abstract concepts and topics of inquiry (the metaparadigm). The science of nursing, on this view, was value-free. The discipline and the practice of nursing share a value orientation, it was argued, but values of practice must influence the discipline only indirectly. The values of the practice determine the topics and concepts of the metaparadigm. Once these topics are chosen, the resulting science is free from their influence. The answer to question (1), then, was that the discipline and practice of nursing are connected at the most abstract level. The metaparadigm reflects the values of the profession, and it directs the research agenda of the discipline.

Questions of philosophy

The dispute over the character of nursing theory in the 1960s and 1970s shows that two further philosophical issues were at stake. One key question was:

3. How do the values that inform nursing practice relate to nursing research and theory?

Practice theorists were committed to the idea that nursing research had to incorporate nursing values. They were criticized on the grounds that proper scientific theory must be value-free. The scientific character of practice theory was also called into question because practice theory did not have the appropriate form. The philosophical question underlying this part of the dispute, then, was:

4. What is the character of scientific theories?

Questions (3) and (4) are central issues in the philosophy of science. The discussion that led up to the consensus of the late 1970s was, strictly speaking, a philosophical debate.

The developments in nursing theory since the 1970s have continued to address these questions. Qualitative research dominated the metatheoretical discussion of the 1980s. Many scholars embraced it not only as a useful methodological tool, but also as a fundamental orientation for the whole discipline. Proponents of qualitative research argued against the idea that science is value-free. They also rejected the idea that inquiry required the discovery of laws. The qualitative research movement thus directly addressed both questions (3) and (4).

In the 1990s, middle-range theory was the new direction for the discipline. This literature does not address the question of value-freedom, but it does take a position on the character of scientific theory. Indeed, as Chapter 2 hinted and Chapter 13 will demonstrate, the origins of middle-range theory were a radical rejection of the 1970s' view of theory structure. In retrospect, it is clear that neither movement succeeded in transforming nursing. In different ways, each got assimilated into the mainstream. Nonetheless, the issues about nursing science to which these scholars were responding remain alive. Therefore, a systematic investigation into the philosophical issues that underlie nursing science is of paramount importance. Before diving into the details of the positions and arguments, however, it might be useful to sketch a preliminary map of the ideas to be discussed.

Science, value, and the nursing standpoint

Qualitative research and value-freedom

The relation of science to value is one area in which philosophical thinking has advanced significantly in the last 30 years. Mid-century philosophers of science largely held that good science must be value-free. Values, it was thought, introduced bias and undermined objectivity. Thomas Kuhn's *Structure of Scientific Revolutions* (Kuhn, [1962] 1970) heralded a turn away from philosophical reconstruction of science to a more historical kind of study. Kuhn and other authors found many ways in which moral or political values had influenced important advances in science. Even if science *ought* to be value-free, it often was not. These arguments were part of the broad critique of logical positivism and related ideas in the philosophy of science. In the 1980s, scholars in a number of fields caught the currents of philosophical change. Qualitative research was among the alternative modes of inquiry proposed during this time. The denial of value-freedom was a rallying cry, and it became one of the distinctive features of the new program.

While qualitative researchers critiqued the ideal of scientific value-freedom, they did not succeed in changing the attitudes of nursing scholars. Chapter 16 will trace the history of qualitative research in nursing. The important upshot is that qualitative research came to be treated as a "paradigm" of nursing research. The idea of a paradigm came from Kuhn ([1962] 1970), and it denoted the complex of theory, values, philosophical commitments, practices, and so on that constituted a research program in science. One of Kuhn's central claims was that paradigms were "incommensurable." A consequence of incommensurability is that criticism between paradigms is impossible. Treating qualitative and quantitative research as different paradigms isolated them, limiting the critique of science that emanated from the qualitative research literature. Quantitative research thus continued to be regarded as value-free, while qualitative research was not.

During the same period, philosophers of science continued to explore questions of scientific objectivity and value-freedom. There is a broad consensus today that value-freedom is not a condition for objectivity. Quite the opposite: as we will see in Part II, it is plausible to think that good scientific research *requires* evaluative commitments. In the philosophy of science, the question has changed from "Is science value-free?" to "How do values become integrated into good scientific inquiry?" and "Under what conditions do value commitments compromise scientific research?" Philosophers of science did not limit their discussion to qualitative research. As a result, they developed models of how values function in science that apply to a broad range of methodological approaches, including those regarded as "quantitative" by nurse scholars. Chapter 5 will work through the arguments from this literature, and it will develop some conceptual tools for thinking about how values function within scientific research.

Standpoint epistemology

Some of the best work on the relationship between science and values has been done by feminist philosophers. "Standpoint epistemology" is a particularly interesting development from the perspective of nursing philosophy. On this view, some social positions have a kind of "epistemic privilege." The classic discussions of this idea have concerned race, class, and gender. Standpoint epistemologists argue that persons who occupy subordinate roles established by race, class, or gender can achieve a less distorted view of the conditions of their oppression. A black domestic worker, for example, needs to be able to understand the social world both from the perspective of her white employers and from her own. As she empties the trash and cleans the sheets, she is in a position to know things about her employers and the social status they occupy that is difficult for them to know about themselves. A political commitment to justice will let her value her role and question the dominant account of society. With appropriate empirical work, she might be able to see her own role from both perspectives. She will come to understand both the benefits her work makes possible as well as the realities of her life that are invisible to her employers. The epistemic privilege of a particular, oppressed social position, then, is the knowledge available when the political commitment is combined with empirical investigation. Standpoint epistemologists thus argue that some kinds of knowledge require commitment to political values.

Something counts as a "standpoint" only if it meets a fairly rigorous set of conditions; not just any body of unique experience will count. Chapters 6 and 7 will argue that the nursing role is such a standpoint. In some ways, this is no surprise. After all, the role of the nurse was strongly influenced by gender, racial, and class roles. Nursing knowledge is different from gendered or racial standpoints because the epistemic privilege of the nurse is not knowledge of the social world, but knowledge of human health. Like the domestic worker, a nurse needs to see the world from two perspectives. She not only needs to understand the physician's point of view on health, but she also needs to tend the patient after the physician has left the room. And, again, like the domestic worker, the unique knowledge available from the nursing standpoint requires an evaluative commitment: a commitment to the value of the client's autonomy, health, and overall well-being, as well as the value of the nursing contribution to the client's healthcare. The fundamental values of nursing are thus part and parcel of nursing knowledge, and nursing knowledge only becomes possible as a result of these commitments.

Feminist standpoint epistemologists often say that inquiry begins from women's lives. Similarly, nursing inquiry (both research and theory development) must begin from nurses' lives. If we are truly committed to the importance and value of nursing, the problems with which we begin must be those that arise out of the nursing encounter. This puts us in a position to rethink the relationship between the discipline and the profession (cf. Question 1). This work will argue that the discipline should not govern the profession. Rather, like the practice theorists, it will argue that research and theory development must be closely tied to the needs of practice. This relationship gives unity to the discipline of nursing (cf. Question 2).

Questions and topics are part of nursing scholarship insofar as they ultimately arise from nursing phenomena (as defined by professional practice) or feedback into the solution to nursing problems. The practice theorists, again, had a view something like this, but they struggled with the next question: Given that the profession unifies the discipline, what unifies the profession? Nurse scholars adopted the idea that the discipline must govern the profession precisely because they needed a way to exclude certain activities as not properly part of the nurses' role. And as we saw above, this was part of the reason for the demise of practice theory. We will need to face this question squarely. We will develop the view that the shape of the profession is partly a political and social question. It is something to be negotiated by nursing organizations in relation to social needs and other health care roles. The intellectual basis for nursing is obviously a relevant consideration in these negotiations. Hence, there is a dynamic relationship between the scope of the profession and the boundaries of the discipline.

Theory, science, and nursing knowledge

The received view of theory

We saw in Chapter 2 how nurse scholars drew key ideas about the form (or "syntax") of scientific theory from mid-century philosophy of science. In the 1970s and 1980s, this conception came to be called as "the received view of theory." Chapter 8 will provide a detailed account of this philosophical perspective. According to the received view, theories are like pyramids. At the top are a small number of very abstract and general laws. These laws define the fundamental concepts of the discipline. Theories at the next level down (middle-range theory) specify the abstract concepts of the most general laws. The laws of middle-range theory are derived from the most general laws by specifying values for the variables and describing the local context. Theories are constructed on a broad foundation of observation, and this is the base of the pyramid. The observations confirm low-level theory, and each level of theory supports the level above it. If a prediction fails, and a low-level theory is disconfirmed, then its failure threatens the levels above.

The notion that scientific theories form a hierarchy has had a pervasive influence on nursing scholarship. It strongly supports the idea that nursing needs a meta-paradigm if it is to be a scientific discipline. It has been a part of the insistence that middle-range theories be conceptually or logically related to grand theories. It has influenced attitudes toward borrowed theory and supported the idea that nursing is a basic science. Chapter 9 will take a close look at the nursing literature and the way in which these philosophical ideas about scientific theory appear in it. As mentioned above, the idea that a theory should be a set of laws also played an important role in the differentiation of qualitative from quantitative research. Commitment to the received view has thus influenced the discussion over whether qualitative and quantitative methods could be combined (or "triangulated"). This will be discussed in Part VI.

Conceptions of theory and its role in science have developed in radical ways since the 1970s. Philosophers of science are no longer compelled by a vision of scientific theory as an axiomatic logical structure. Chapter 10 will articulate the reasons why this view of theory and related doctrines were rejected by philosophers of science. One important consequence is that a discipline may be scientific without having theories at a high level of abstraction and generality. Once the philosophical blinders are taken away, it becomes clear that using middle-range theories to apply high-level theories is the exception, not the rule in the sciences. These changes in philosophical conceptions of scientific theory have profound consequences for the way that nurse scholars should think about science.

Explanatory coherence and inter-level models

A philosophical successor to the received view of theory is the "explanatory coherence" view of theory, and this position will be developed in Chapter 12. The metaphor for theories associated with the received view is a pyramid. The explanatory coherence view, by contrast, imagines theories as webs. Around the edge, the theory links to the world through observation. In the web, each strand is supported by its links to others, and these links run both to the edge (observation) and to other parts of the web (other theories). If any part fails, other parts compensate. What makes the web strong is the coherence of the whole, not the strength of any particular part. On an explanatory coherence view of theory, then, a discipline might be entirely composed of mutually supporting bodies of theory at roughly the same level of generality. Anthropology, epidemiology, and neuroscience are good examples of disciplines with this kind of structure. Of course, the idea that a discipline could be composed of a cluster of theories raises the question of unity again. The ideas of the foregoing section provide an answer: the discipline of nursing is unified by the nursing standpoint. Theories are appropriately part of the nursing discipline insofar as they help respond to the needs of professional practice.

Another interesting development in recent philosophy of science has been an emphasis on mechanistic models. Mid-century philosophy of science was fascinated by examples like Newtonian physics, where a small number of laws explained a large number of phenomena. In the 1980s and 1990s, philosophers of science came to realize that other scientific domains did not develop the same kinds of theory. In areas like biochemistry, molecular genetics, or neuroscience, scientists worked with models, not theories. Models decompose a phenomenon into elements, and show how those parts work together to create the observed behavior. The object is not to discover laws that apply to a wide range of phenomena. Rather, the object is to create a model that lets the scientist predict how changes to the elements will affect the outcomes.

Thinking about science as model building, rather than theory testing, made a brief, but significant appearance in the nursing literature. Chapter 2 noted how Suppe contributed to the early work on middle-range theory. Chapter 13 will develop Suppe's ideas (and related work) in more detail. Once we remove middle-range theory from the idea that theory must be arranged in a hierarchy, we can see a fresh importance to Suppe's work. Inter-level models, for example, are one useful form of middle-range theory. Inter-level models explain how phenomena at one level (e.g., the experience of pain) can be related to a system at another (e.g., neural circuits). This sort of knowledge can be crucial for patient care. If nursing knowledge aims to respond to problems visible from the nursing standpoint, developing inter-level models should be central to nursing inquiry.

Consequences for nursing knowledge

Commitment to a hierarchical conception of theory influenced nurse scholars' attitudes toward borrowed theory. Genuine nursing inquiry could not proceed, it was argued, by using theory borrowed from other disciplines. Since the highest level laws and concepts gave meaning to the lower level, middle-range theories could not be removed from their disciplinary homes. Once we have worked through the philosophical issues about theory structure and conceptual content, there will be philosophical space for a different attitude toward borrowed theory. Concepts do get their content from context, but contexts are not hermetically sealed. Theories at low levels of abstraction are oriented toward particular kinds of phenomena, and they respect no disciplinary boundaries. This means that there is no philosophical barrier to borrowing theories from other domains. Moreover, on an explanatory coherence view of theory and confirmation, the discipline of nursing is epistemically strengthened when its theories are linked to others. Finally, if the discipline is unified by the nursing standpoint, borrowing theory presents no threat to the discipline of nursing. A theory is appropriately used by nurse scholars insofar as it helps solve nursing problems. It does not matter who first developed the theory or what the original purpose might have been.

Nurse scholars' understanding of the relationship between qualitative and quantitative research has also been influenced by the prevailing view of theory. As noted above, qualitative researchers embraced the critique of the received view of theory. As the debate progressed, however, the critical power of the ideas was contained by isolating qualitative research. Qualitative and quantitative research came to be treated as distinct paradigms, each with its own theory structures, forms of evidence, and philosophical presuppositions. Qualitative research ironically came to reinforce the power of the received view of theory. What the philosophical critique of the received view showed, however, is that *quantitative* theory had been misconceived. Quantitative research also involves theories that are holistic, value laden, and contextual. Once the force of the critique has been appreciated, the sharp line between qualitative and quantitative research disappears. Part IV will argue that "qualitative" and "quantitative" characterize research methods, not paradigms. As such, they are not fundamental commitments of researchers. Rather, they are methodological choices to be made in the light of the research questions and prior knowledge about the subject of study.

Conclusion: closing the gap

In a practice discipline like nursing, a relevance gap is profoundly troubling. In Chapter 2, we saw how the relevance gap opened because of the answers to philosophical questions about nursing. The consensus view makes nursing research and theory development independent of the needs of practice. To bring theory and practice together again, we need to rethink the philosophy. Doing so will invoke controversy, but there is no alternative. The only way to close the relevance gap is to articulate ideas that are at odds with the current consensus. This chapter has sketched a way of answering the philosophical questions about nursing science in a systematically different way. Both nurse scholars and philosophers have provided arguments to support these contentions, but the point of this chapter has not been to present those arguments. Rather, it has been to illustrate how research and theory development can be linked much more closely to the needs of the profession. On the standpoint view, relevance to nursing practice becomes a criterion for inclusion in the nursing discipline. We can return to Reed and Lawrence's view that nursing knowledge must be useful and significant to practicing nurses (Reed & Lawrence, 2008, p. 423). The philosophical view sketched here thus has a chance of closing the relevance gap. That possibility alone makes the details worth considering.

Part II
Values and the Nursing Standpoint

Introduction to Part II

Professional nursing is a moral calling. Discussions of the nursing profession emphasize the importance of empirical knowledge, but surely the moral basis of the profession is equally significant. And the moral dimension of the profession is not limited to the problems of bioethics. Caring for others—whether by a professional nurse or by a parent, friend, or lover—is a way of morally responding to them. There is, then, a moral dimension to the core mission of nursing. Nursing has a social mandate, and this means that the profession has political dimensions too. In the professional practice of nursing there is a deep, organic relationship between nursing knowledge and nursing values. Any nursing intervention has to be based both on what is known about the situation and what is good, right, or valuable. In the discipline, however, the relationship between nursing knowledge and nursing ethics or politics has not been so clear. Indeed, the history of nursing shows that the relationship between the professional values and disciplinary knowledge has often been problematic.

The relationship between nursing values and nursing theories has been an important part in nursing debates about theory. Chapter 3 suggested that adopting a different view of how nursing values are related to nursing science might change the relationship between theory and practice, and thereby help close the relevance gap. This Part will consider the issues about values in more detail. In the 1970s, nurse scholars found ways to let values influence the scope of nursing science, and yet keep the content of the science value-free. Chapter 4 will present the debate within nursing as it has unfolded since the late 1960s. During that period, philosophers began to question whether good science must be value-free. Chapter 5 will work through the philosophical issues. Philosophers of science today commonly hold that that science requires value-judgments. The important questions are: What values? And what role do they play in inquiry? Chapter 5 is somewhat technical, but its aim is to develop a philosophical framework for thinking about how values are related to scientific inquiry. Chapter 6 will take a close look at the values of professional nursing and how they influence the discipline. It will argue that nursing knowledge is best understood as a kind of standpoint epistemology. Because of the professional role of nurses, nursing has the potential to develop a more complete, less distorted understanding of human health. Chapter 7 will develop this idea and begin to explore its ramifications for nursing knowledge.

In many ways, the work of Chapters 6 and 7 is foundational for the rest of this book. They develop the idea that nursing has the capacity to develop unique knowledge about human health *in virtue of nursing's socially determined role*. The importance of nursing practice in nursing knowledge has been obscured by philosophical ideas about science. Part III will begin to strip away some of the inadequate preconceptions, and Parts IV and V will start to articulate a conception of nursing science that is responsive to the nursing standpoint.

Practice values and the disciplinary knowledge base

Nurse scholars have long recognized that the moral dimension of nursing needs to be connected to its research dimension. The practice theorists, introduced in Chapter 2, were the first nursing scholars to have a well worked out idea about how professional values related to the disciplinary knowledge. Dickoff and James, in particular, developed a view of nursing theory that had an explicit place for inquiry into nursing values. Practice theory was criticized on this point, and the current consensus about science and values results from those arguments. To understand the current views about how the values of practice inform nursing research, then, we need to look carefully at the arguments and their history within nursing.

Dickoff and James' practice theory

To incorporate values within scientific theory, Dickoff and James began with a rather broad definition of a theory: "a conceptual system or framework invented to some purpose" (Dickoff & James, 1968, p. 198). Their intention was to assimilate a wide range of nursing research activities within the scope of "theory." Nursing scholarship in the 1960s was concerned, among other things, to find ways of articulating and testing the knowledge that was implicit in practice. Dickoff and James's definition of theory was broad enough to bring such work within the scope of proper theorizing.

Dickoff and James identified four levels of theory, and argued that each had its own purposes and criteria of evaluation. The purpose of the first level (what they called "factor-isolating theories") was to articulate a set of concepts (factors) that were important in a given domain. At this level, phenomena are identified, named, and distinguished, but no relations expressed or generalizations made.[1] The second level of situation-depicting theory uses the basic concepts to create descriptions. The difference between the first and second levels is analogous to the difference between the words "pain," "cancer," and "patient," on the one hand, and sentences such as "this patient has cancer," or "some cancer patients have severe pain" on the other. The first level is no more than a list of words; nothing is said with these words. Only at the second level are the concepts related and testable statements made. Dickoff and James use anatomy and natural history as examples of theories at the second level, and one can imagine that much of contemporary epidemiological research would fall into this category. Causal relationships (e.g., "cancer causes pain") were to be articulated at the third level of theorizing, what they called "situation-relating theories." In their description of this level of theory, Dickoff and James defer to the mid-century philosophers of science (Dickoff & James, 1968). The first three levels of theory, then, are designed to encompass all theorizing in the (nonprofessional) scientific disciplines.

While the first three levels of theory are found in the natural and social sciences, according to Dickoff and James, the profession of nursing required something more. The knowledge base of the profession cannot be limited to descriptions or causal relationships. Nurses have to know what to do, and this requires knowing that the goal to be achieved is a *good* one. Therefore, Dickoff and James conclude that professional nursing needs a conceptual apparatus with the purpose of directing action toward appropriate goals (Dickoff et al., 1968a, p. 555). This was captured by the highest level of theory, what they called "situation-producing theory." Situation-producing theory is therefore normative in the sense that it identifies what makes certain forms of the activity good or excellent. It specifies the goals of nursing. In addition, a situation-producing theory must say how the goals may be reached. This requires a description and analysis of the relevant parts of the practice and of the practice environment that would be captured in the first two levels of theory. Situation-producing theory would also require showing how those activities should be organized so as to achieve the goals of the practice. Hence, a situation-producing theory must rely on causal generalizations too (third level theory). In this way, situation-producing theory depends on prior development and testing of theories at all of the lower levels (Dickoff & James, 1968; Dickoff et al., 1968a). But it goes further, for situation-producing theory must also articulate the goals and goods of nursing practice, and show how they can be achieved.

Values and theory testing

Because situation-producing theory includes values, there are important questions about how it might be tested. Dickoff and James describe situation-producing

---

[1] This seems to presuppose that concepts can be given meaning prior to the development of theories. There is good reason to reject this idea, and Chapter 14 will articulate some of the arguments. The critique to be canvassed has important consequences for the practice of concept analysis in nursing; see Rodgers (1989, [1993] 2000), Paley (1996), and Risjord (2009).

theory in terms of means and ends (or goals). A goal is an outcome that the nurse *ought* to strive for. It is something good for the patient (or the nurse). To decide that something is a goal is therefore a value-judgment. Now, one distinctive feature of value-judgments is that they are not directly testable. A statement like "murder is morally wrong" is not shown to be false by describing the murder rate in New York City. This is a general problem for all forms of theory that incorporate values: What kind of evidence might be used to test them? On what grounds should we accept or reject a situation-producing theory?

Dickoff and James provided elaborate descriptions of the elements of a situation-producing theory, but they said very little about how such theories might be tested. When Dickoff and James were writing, very few nursing interventions had been tested. A study that must[2] have figured in Dickoff and James's thinking was "The effect of nursing on the incidence of postoperative vomiting" by Dumas and Leonard (1963). This work set out to test the hypothesis that "the use of a particular nursing approach in the care of surgical patients would reduce the incidence of postoperative vomiting" (Dumas & Leonard, 1963, p. 12). The study used Orlando's *The Dynamic Nurse-Patient Relationship* (1961) to design the intervention, and Orlando's work fit the definition of a situation-producing theory. In the intervention, the nurse talked with the patient about his or her anxiety about the approaching operation and tried to relieve it. The control group received standard nursing care, which at the time did not include a discussion about the impending procedure. The study found that the nursing intervention had a significant effect.

Notice how Dumas and Leonard's study incorporated nursing goals and values. The intended outcome was to reduce postoperative vomiting, and this is a desirable goal. It is a specific instance of the more general goal of relieving the patient's emotional distress, which was something that Orlando had proposed as an important objective for nursing. Even more generally, Orlando's work promoted the patient's psychological well-being as a central value. This study, then, was a vivid example of how a "situation-producing theory" might be subject to empirical test.

Dickoff and James explain their view about how situation-producing theory should be tested in their essay "Theory in a practice discipline part II: practice oriented research" (1968b). There, they say that situation-producing theories must be "coherent," "palatable," and "feasible" (Dickoff *et al.*, 1968b, p. 670). The theory is coherent if it can bring about the specified end. The postoperative vomiting study seems to have been aiming to show that the theory is "coherent" in Dickoff and James's sense. The experiment was set up to determine whether the intervention brought about the goal of reducing postoperative vomiting. A situation-producing theory is "feasible" insofar as the implementation of the prescribed practices fits the needs and constraints of the institutional environment. The postoperative vomiting study does little to show feasibility. For all we know from the study, the kind of counseling given by the nurse in the study is too time consuming to be practical in the busy environment of an ICU. Of course, the study was not designed to

[2] The second author of this paper, Robert Leonard, was closely associated with Yale School of Nursing and the development of practice theory (cf. Wald & Leonard, 1964).

show feasibility; such demonstrations would require further research. The question of "palatability" is whether the goal, when achieved, is still desirable. Reduction of postoperative vomiting seems like a positive outcome, but we could be wrong. For example, suppose that the patients in the study found that refraining from vomiting would leave them feeling nauseous and anxious for a long time, while vomiting was only momentarily unpleasant. The apparently desirable goal of reducing vomiting would thus have been shown to be not so good after all.

Challenges to Dickoff and James' criteria

There are several problems with Dickoff and James's conception of how value-laden theories might be tested. First, any determination of palatability would require appeal to further values. In other words, an outcome could only be judged valuable (or not), in the light of other values. For example, if reducing postoperative vomiting were "unpalatable," then there must have been something else more valuable that was lost when this result was achieved. And if the result were palatable, it must be that the reduction of postoperative vomiting fit with other values that were prominent in the situation. At best, then, palatability is a test of whether the actual outcome of the intervention coheres with all of the other values in play. When we recognize that palatability is another kind of coherence, it becomes clear that a study such as Dumas and Leonard's is only part of what is required to demonstrate palatability. The study shows us that postoperative vomiting can be reduced by a particular intervention. Whether that result is good depends on a further argument that presupposes a cluster of nursing goals, goods, and values.

The Dumas and Leonard's study seems intended to demonstrate that the goals of Orlando's theory can be achieved, but there are difficulties here too. Among Orlando's stated goals of nursing is the "direct responsibility to see that the patient's needs for help are met" (Orlando, 1961, p. 29). To meet the patient's needs, the nurse:

"(1) *initiates a process of helping the patient express the specific meaning of his behavior in order to ascertain his distress and (2) helps the patient explore the distress in order to ascertain the help he requires so that his distress maybe relieved."* (Orlando, 1961, p. 29)

Dumas and Leonard designed the experimental treatment to implement the means suggested by Orlando. Their protocol required that:

"(a) *the nurse explores with the patient her observations of his behavior to determine whether he is experiencing distress. (b) The nurse explores further to find out what is causing the distress and to determine what is needed to relieve the distress. (c) The nurse uses the information elicited in the first two steps to select an appropriate course of action to relieve the distress. Following this action, (d) the nurse checks with the patient to ascertain whether this course of action did in fact relieve the patient's distress. If the patient's verbal and non-verbal behavior convinces the nurse that the distress is relieved, the process is completed. Otherwise, the process begins all over again."* (Dumas & Leonard, 1963, p. 12)

The study showed that this intervention has an effect, when compared with no intervention at all. In the narrow sense of Dickoff and James's "coherence," the study shows coherence: the goal of reducing postoperative vomiting (which is presumably one of the patient's needs) can be achieved by this intervention. However, it gives very little empirical justification for Orlando's theory as a whole. That is, it provides little or no evidence to believe that Orlando's theory is correct, true, or accurate.[3] Since it is Orlando's theory that is value-laden, not the specific intervention, the Dumas and Leonard's study does little to show how value-laden theory might be tested.

Considered as a test of Orlando's theory, there are two further deficiencies in Dumas and Leonard's study. First, the experimental contrast is rather coarse. The control group was given no nursing support:

> *"The control patients were carried to the operating room by an orderly and were not accompanied by a nurse. They waited alone in the corridor until time to be put on the operating table."* (Dumas & Leonard, 1963, pp. 12–13)

This procedure seems guaranteed to raise anxiety. Hence, for all we know, any conversation with a concerned party—whether or not it explored the source of the anxiety—might have been equally effective. To demonstrate that the specific features of the intervention bring about the outcome, the study needs more sophisticated controls. For example, a control group with whom the nurse simply made small talk would have helped show that the effect was due to the content of the discussion, not just the human contact.

A further problem is that there was a rather weak relationship between the protocol and Orlando's theory. It is not clear, for example, whether the needs will be met by getting the specific help desired (e.g., an explanation of the procedure, another pillow, or a glass of water) or through the conversation. To put the point another way, any test of a theory should be set up so that if the test *fails*, then some change to the theory is mandated. If Leonard and Dumas had found that their intervention had no effect, it is not clear what, if any, impact there would be on Orlando's theory. The relationship between the theory and the intervention is just too vague.

Beckstrand's critique

Fact and value

The foregoing challenges to practice theory all concern the way in which practice theories might be tested or justified, and they arise from the way that practice

---

[3] The criticism in this paragraph should not be understood as diminishing the importance of this study. It was one of the very first attempts to test an intervention based on nursing scholarship. It was very important as a demonstration that the discipline of nursing had the potential to develop the profession's knowledge base.

theory blends descriptive and evaluative statements. Beckstrand argued on philosophical grounds against the very idea of practice theory as a distinct kind of theory (Beckstrand, 1978a, 1978b, 1980). Beckstrand began her argument with the claim that scientific knowledge is entirely descriptive: "Science is concerned with identifying lawlike empirical relations, with confirming or corroborating their factual nature, with describing and explaining them, and with determining their interrelationships and empirical consequences" (Beckstrand, 1978a, p. 606). Citing Hempel (1965), Nagel (1961), and Popper (1968)—all major figures in mid-century philosophy of science—she emphasized the role of laws in scientific theorizing. She recognized that applying science to practice can be difficult, messy, and uncertain. Nonetheless, nursing practice must use knowledge of causally necessary and sufficient conditions to achieve its ends.

Beckstrand agreed with the practice theorists that nursing practice involved a variety of value-judgments. Moral value determines what actions a nurse ought (or ought not) to perform and what kinds of virtues she ought to cultivate. Questions of moral value and obligation are answered by ethical theories. While she does not dwell on the difference, Beckstrand took ethical theories to be utterly different from scientific theories. Ethical theories articulate "standards for evaluation," while scientific theories describe and explain the natural (and human) world. Practice theory purported to blend description and evaluation within one, special kind of theory. Beckstrand argued that, on the contrary, the knowledge required by practitioners was the simple conjunction of scientific theories and ethical theories.

Intrinsic and instrumental values

Beckstrand recognized that the strongest case for practice theory was the "nonmoral" value-judgments that figure in nursing practice:

> *"Here, one is concerned with the ascription of the qualities of goodness and badness on nonmoral grounds to things like cars, hospital care, and movies; the outcomes or results of actions like nursing interventions; and to people and their traits."* (Beckstrand, 1978a, p. 610)

In these examples, it is difficult to neatly separate the factual and evaluative components. They therefore seem to support the idea that there must be a special form of value-laden theory. The judgment that a nursing intervention is good is clearly a value-judgment, but it is equally clear that such a judgment also depends on empirical (scientific) knowledge. This was just Dickoff and James' point. Beckstrand attacks this problem by distinguishing "instrumental" from "intrinsic" values. Instrumental values are things that are good because they help achieve some end or goal, and their value depends on that goal. For example, if I need to repair my shirt, a needle and thread are valuable. If, by contrast, I do not care whether my clothing is torn, then the needle and thread have no value for me. Instrumental values are thus relative in a sense; their value is relative to the chosen goal. Goals, on the other hand, are different. They are not always valuable merely as a means to something else. Their value is intrinsic.[4]

Having distinguished instrumental from intrinsic values, Beckstrand followed Hempel (1965) in arguing that whether something has instrumental value is a *scientific* question:

> *"According to Hempel, an instrumental judgment of value asserts either that [a course of action] M is a (definitely or probably) sufficient means for attaining the end or goal G, or that it is a (definitely or probably) necessary means for attaining it.*
>
> *This means that the knowledge of instrumental value is scientific knowledge, and it can be used in practice in the same way."* (Beckstrand, 1978a, p. 611)

Questions of instrumental value, according to Hempel, are questions about sufficient or necessary conditions: Does the chosen means bring about the goal? Is it required for attaining the goal? If so, then the means is instrumentally valuable (relative to the goal). As Beckstrand argued, science is concerned with discovering generalizations about causally necessary or sufficient conditions. Knowledge of instrumental values is thus scientific knowledge. Intrinsic values, on the other hand, are valuable in themselves, and scientific theory will not tell us what is intrinsically valuable. Knowledge of intrinsic value requires ethical theory. Nonmoral value-judgments, such as the judgment that a nursing intervention is good, therefore decompose into two parts: ethical and empirical.

To see the consequences of Beckstrand's distinction between instrumental and intrinsic values, consider the postoperative vomiting study again. Orlando takes the reduction of patient distress to be an intrinsic good. It is something at which nursing action aims, and it is not valuable as a means to anything else. Whether reducing patient distress is really valuable, according to Beckstrand, would be a question for ethical theory. Once we have determined (via ethical theorizing) that reduction of patient distress is a goal for which nurses should strive, we can ask what means will achieve this goal. Dumas and Leonard make the reasonable assumption that vomiting is distressing, hence reducing vomiting will reduce patient distress. The questions then become scientific: Will this or that intervention reduce postoperative vomiting? What seemed to be a special kind of theory therefore reduces to ethical theory (determining the goals of nursing) and scientific theory (determining the means).

Carper's fact–value distinction

Beckstrand's separation of scientific knowledge from ethical knowledge paralleled Carper's patterns of knowing (Carper, 1978). It was through Carper's famous essay

---

[4] Of course, a goal may be proximate. Thus, I may value the needle and thread to repair my shirt, but the goal of repairing my shirt is itself valuable as a means to some further goal, like presenting myself well at a job interview. Many have argued that, on pain of regress, not all values can be instrumental. There must be some values that are intrinsic.

that the strict separation of scientific knowledge and ethical knowledge was promulgated among nurse scholars. Based on a survey and analysis of nursing scholarship through the mid-1970s, Carper suggested that nursing knowledge could be analyzed into four domains or "patterns":

> *"(a) empirics, the science of nursing; (b) esthetics, the art of nursing; (c) the component of personal knowledge in nursing; and (d) ethics, the component of moral knowledge in nursing."* (Carper, 1978, p. 14)

While there is much to say about the aesthetic and personal knowledge patterns, our concern here is with the ethical and empiric patterns. "Empirics" was intended to encompass the scientific side of nursing. Carper's conception of empirics is virtually identical to Beckstrand's conception of scientific knowledge: "knowledge that is systematically organized into general laws and theories for the purpose of describing, explaining, and predicting phenomena of special concern to the discipline of nursing" (Carper, 1978, p. 14). Carper's description of ethical knowledge is also similar to Beckstrand's. She emphasizes the role of ethical theories in justifying moral decisions in nursing. While she does not distinguish between moral and nonmoral values, or intrinsic and instrumental values, she does include knowledge of the goals of nursing within the ethical domain. Like Beckstrand, then, Carper reduces the apparently value-laden knowledge necessary for nursing practice to scientific knowledge (empirics) and ethical knowledge.

Carper's analysis of nursing knowledge and Beckstrand's direct criticism combined to eclipse practice theory in nursing. In her essay "Contemporary nursing research: its Relevance for nursing practice," Fawcett explicitly brought both essays to bear on Dickoff and James's contention that professional nursing required situation-producing theory. After showing how nursing research could be fit within the first three levels of Dickoff and James's hierarchy, she argued that "special knowledge, or prescriptive theory, is not needed by the practitioner" (Fawcett, 1983, p. 173). Carper's empirical pattern encompassed the basic science of nursing, and the ethical pattern provided the professional values. By the early 1980s, then, the mainstream of nursing scholarship held that nursing practice was best served by thinking of nursing in terms of separate empirical and ethical patterns of knowing.

Problems with patterns

The disintegration of nursing knowledge

There are a number of difficulties with the way Beckstrand and Carper pulled nursing values out of nursing science. One of the striking features of Carper's essay is that once the patterns are distinguished, they are not reintegrated. To be sure, she does say that the patterns are "separate but interrelated and interdependent." But in the same sentence she goes on to say that each pattern should be "taught and understood according to its distinctive logic, the restricted circumstances in which it is valid, the kinds of data it subsumes and the methods by which each particular kind of truth is distinguished and warranted" (Carper, 1978, p. 22). This body of differentia—logic, circumstances of validity, data, and methods—are profound epistemic differences. While Carper's statement that the patterns are interrelated and independent is no doubt correct, it is difficult to see how the interrelationship could be achieved. It is not enough to assert that the patterns are interrelated, as many authors do; we need an account of how they are related. We will return to this point below.

The obfuscation of evaluative commitments

While treating knowledge of fact and knowledge of value as independent seems to introduce some philosophical clarity and rigor, Michael Yeo argued that, to the contrary, "it is conceptually muddled and highly misleading to divide nursing theories into those that are valuational (normative) and those that are descriptive (scientific)" (Yeo, 1989, p. 190). Yeo drew this conclusion from a close reading of Roy's adaptation model. That model, he argued, is shot through with value commitments:

> *"The term managing stimuli, for example, which Roy has lately adopted for describing nursing intervention, is not without important value assumptions and implications. The management metaphor conceptualizes the nurse as in some sense having a superior role in the nurse-patient relationship: the nurse manages, the patient adapts".* (Yeo, 1989, p. 35)

The evaluative dimension of the phrase "managing stimuli" is directly relevant to the way that a practicing nurse comports herself. Yet, since it is not the sort of idea that would appear in ethical theories, it gets treated as if it were a flat, scientific description. This "conceptual muddle" becomes "highly misleading" when it serves to hide the moral (or political) commitments of Roy's theory. The moral dimensions of "managing stimuli" are not made explicit, and therefore they are not scrutinized. In the case of Roy's model, Yeo argued, this gives rise to an inconsistency between her explicit affirmation of the patient's voice, and the implicit suppression of that voice by the other terms of the model.

Pamela Reed argued more broadly that:

> *"There are many nursing phenomena that, when conceptualized for research, stimulate if not demand ethical reflection by the theorist. Personal biases and assumptions about emotional illness, adolescent development, and female sexuality, for example, which typically elicit presumptive notions about the value of time, independence, and other assumed goods can have moral influences on the types of conceptualization constructed in the study of the phenomena as they relate to health".* (Reed, 1989, p. 6)

Like Yeo, Reed argued that ethical reflection is a necessary component of empirical inquiry in nursing. Similar points have been made by other nurse scholars (Tinkle & Beaton, 1983; Browne, 2001; Kirkham & Anderson, 2002). Treating empirics and ethics as separate but (somehow) related patterns obscures the way in which nursing science requires moral or political evaluation.

The role of theory in ethical knowledge

A further kind of problem with the way that Carper and Beckstrand treat ethics is that they overemphasize the role that ethical theories play in ethical knowledge. They think that ethical theories and scientific theories are parallel sorts of knowledge. For example, a nurse may come to believe that her patient's heart rate is dangerously erratic through applying her theoretical knowledge of pulmonary physiology. Or again, a nurse might use the Kübler–Ross theory to interpret her patient's angry remarks as a stage of the grieving process. In these cases, details about the individual case are added to the generalizations of the theory to make inferences about the patient. Carper and Beckstrand seem to think that knowledge of ethical codes or standards has a similar relation to moral judgment.

The idea that ethical judgment follows from theory was recently reinforced by Fawcett *et al.* (2001), where each of Carper's patterns is treated as a kind of theory. According to Fawcett and her colleagues, the theories within the ethical pattern of knowing are standards of practice and codes of ethics (Fawcett *et al.*, 2001, p. 116). On this model, for example, a nurse would know that she should not medicate a competent patient who has refused treatment because she knows that, according to the American Nurses Association Code of Ethics (2009), patients have the right to refuse treatment. However, as Yeo remarked, "If one has to derive one's respect for autonomy from an ethical theory, one is in deep trouble" (Yeo, 1989, p. 192).

David Seedhouse called the idea that ethical theories or codes will tell us how to act the "ethics myth" (Seedhouse, 2000, p. 178). Seedhouse argues that ethical theories are too abstract and general to provide specific guidance. We cannot reach ethical decisions by simply adding the details of the case to an ethical theory in the way that values are inserted into a mathematical equation. The real work of ethical reasoning is not a matter of applying general ideas to specific cases, but becoming sensitive to the morally salient dimensions of a situation. Ethical codes are expressions of professional commitment. They guide us by highlighting areas of moral concern. Arguably, then, ethical theories have a different relationship to our ethical judgments than scientific theories have to our empirical beliefs. The problem with Beckstrand and Carper, not to mention Fawcett *et al.*, is that they misplace the role of theory in ethical judgment.

The difference between ethical theories and scientific theories highlights a further aspect of Yeo's remarks about "managing stimuli" (Yeo, 1989, p. 189). His argument was that empirical theories have hidden value commitments. Yeo's discussion of "managing stimuli" showed that the concepts of nursing theory can have meanings that are partly evaluative and partly descriptive. Fully understanding the ethical parts of nursing knowledge, then, requires making explicit and reflecting on the evaluative character of terms such as "managing stimuli" or "patient distress." Ethical codes provide little or no guidance because they must work with concepts that are not bound to specific theories, communities, or places (Seedhouse, 2000, p. 5). Ethical theory, as traditionally conceived within philosophy, is concerned to understand concepts such as good, right, justice, equality, autonomy, or beneficence. It has little or nothing to say about the concrete evaluations that are embedded within specific research programs. Splitting nursing knowledge into an empirical pattern and an ethical pattern, then, not only prevents us from appreciating the deeper moral consequences of nursing research but also robs us of tools for articulating these consequences.

Sociopolitical knowing

A similar problem with separating knowledge of fact and knowledge of value into separate patterns is raised by Jill White's discussion of "sociopolitical knowing" (White, 1995). White argued that it was important for nurses to be politically engaged with larger social issues.[5] This is a part of nursing's social mandate, and social issues such as poverty, unemployment, and drug addiction impinge directly on areas of nursing concern. She suggested that the patterns of knowing be expanded to include a fifth pattern, the "sociopolitical pattern" of knowing:

> *"Sociopolitical knowing may be conceptualized as including understandings on two levels: (1) the sociopolitical context of the persons (nurse and patient) and (2) the sociopolitical context of nursing as a practice profession, including both society's understanding of nursing and nursing's understanding of society and its politics."* (White, 1995, p. 256)

Notice that the levels in White's characterization are both descriptive and factual. Knowledge of the sociopolitical context of nursing is the result of research in history and sociology, and these are empirical disciplines. It is clear from White's discussion, however, that the sociopolitical pattern is supposed to be normative as well. The sociopolitical pattern involves commitment to political causes, advocacy, and engagement in political debate. Thus, empirical knowledge of the sociopolitical context is not enough; sociopolitical knowing requires both factual knowledge and political (or moral) commitment. Once this is recognized, however, it calls the status of the proposed sociopolitical pattern into question. Is the sociopolitical pattern really a fifth pattern of knowing? Or is it a combination of the empiric pattern and the ethical pattern? If Beckstrand's argument against practice theory is sound, then it applies to sociopolitical knowing too.

White's discussion of the sociopolitical pattern shows how it resists analysis into ethical and empirical patterns. She wrote:

> *"Violence, drug dependence, and diabetes are examples of responses to what are inherently political rather than simply personal problems, and nurses' efforts to deal with them require nurses to articulate what they see as resulting from societies' structures."* (White, 1995, p. 256)

Dealing with drug dependence, for instance, will require knowledge of the physiology and psychology of addiction, the sociology of the drug culture, and so on. This

---

[5] Afaf Meleis made similar arguments in a number of publications, for example (Meleis, 1987, 1992; Meleis & Im, 1998). Her view will be discussed and developed in Chapter 11.

is empirical knowledge, but it presupposes the ethical or political judgment that drug dependence is a social problem. Our understanding of the moral and political dimensions of drug dependence frames and informs the empirical research on it. We seek to understand the physiology of addiction because we want to find ways of mitigating its effects on individuals and on society. Our philosophical commitment to autonomy colors our understanding of the physiology. Similar points go for the other social and political problems to which nurses respond. Nursing knowledge must integrate ethical and political judgment with empirical science.

While the knowledge required for responding to social and political problems resists analysis into ethical and empirical patterns, it is not clear that adding a fifth pattern is the best response. There are reasons to resist White's suggestion that we recognize a fifth pattern. The fundamental problem with Carper's patterns of knowing is that there is no account of how the patterns are to be related. As we have already seen, the literature insists that the patterns are part of a single whole, but nothing has been said about how the integration works. When we introduce a fifth pattern, the question of the relationship among patterns arises again. How is the knowledge in the empiric pattern related to the knowledge in the sociopolitical pattern? Postulating yet another pattern to mediate the empiric and the sociopolitical patterns would be to start a vicious regress. No, the problem lies in the isolation of the patterns in the first place. Carper's essay was important because it showed the variety of forms of knowledge that professional nursing required. The mistake was to reify these different aspects of knowledge into separate patterns, each with its own logic, circumstances of validity, data, and methods.

Conclusion: fact and value in nursing knowledge

The discipline of nursing cannot abide a strict and absolute distinction between scientific knowledge and ethical/political knowledge. Both White's discussion of the political side of nursing knowledge and Yeo's arguments about the moral and political presuppositions of nursing theories suggest that nursing knowledge must be both normative and descriptive. At the same time, Carper and Beckstrand pointed out some very important differences between scientific and ethical theories, both in terms of their justification and their content. The need to integrate these differences gives rise to some profound challenges. If nursing theories incorporate value commitments, how can scientific methods test them? Dickoff and James had an answer to this question, but as we saw above, it was not entirely successful. Furthermore, the integration of ethics and politics into science is often troublesome. How can nursing science lay claim to objectivity, if we refuse to isolate and extract the evaluative commitments? To answer these questions, we need to draw on some philosophical resources.

Models of value-laden science

A quick argument seems to establish that values have no role in science: science tells us how things are, not how they ought to be; evaluations say only how things ought to be; therefore, science must be value-free. In addition, when moral or political values do play a role in science, they sometimes serve to bias and distort the results. We have had too much experience with drug companies suppressing negative results or politicians editing scientific reports to fully trust value-laden science. At the same time, values are difficult to expunge from science. As we saw in Chapter 4, values sneak in unexpectedly. As a result, the questions of whether and how science can be value-laden have been vivid in the philosophy of science.

In mid-twentieth century philosophy of science, the dominant view was that value-laden science could not be objective. During the latter half of the twentieth century, a number of philosophical arguments undermined this position. While it would not be correct to say that there are *no* defenders of strict value-freedom, the pendulum has swung to the opposite extreme. Most philosophers of science agree that values do (or even, must) play a role in science. The important questions in contemporary philosophy of science are: What role(s) do values play in good science? Under what conditions do values introduce bias? And how can value-laden science be epistemically sound? For the purposes of this work, we do not need fully general answers to all of these questions. Rather, we will draw on and develop some of the existing philosophical work so as to create a more robust understanding of the value-laden character of nursing knowledge.

The Johnson model: nursing values as guides for theory

Chapter 4 argued that the strict separation between the empirical and moral/political aspects of nursing knowledge was untenable. Nursing science is informed by the value-commitments implicit in nursing practice. The problem with

Beckstrand's and Carper's essays was that they had no model of how empirical and ethical knowledge might be related. There is, however, a model in the nursing literature that maintains the distinction between empirical and ethical knowledge, yet explains how they interact. It was presented first in Johnson's "Development of theory: a requisite for nursing as a primary health profession" (Johnson, 1974) and developed by Donaldson and Crowley in "The discipline of nursing" (Donaldson & Crowley, 1978).

These nurse scholars all begin with nursing's social mandate. Nurses have a role in health care and are charged with certain responsibilities because they can provide a socially valuable service. The scope of nursing practice is thus partly a social and political question, but not entirely. Nurses are entrusted with responsibility in a particular domain because they have relevant, specialized knowledge. As we saw in Chapters 1 and 2, the perceived need for an expertise unique to nursing made developing the nursing research enterprise a high priority for nurses. Given the scope of nursing expertise, the proper boundaries of nursing action could be set. In this sense, the discipline of nursing would "govern" the professional practice of nursing (Donaldson & Crowley, 1978, p. 118).

The social mandate gives the nursing profession a value orientation. The mandate for nursing is directly influenced by the commitments of leaders who shape the health care institutions. Roles for nurses within the larger health care system are negotiated, and these roles presuppose that certain kinds of goals need to be achieved. The social value of the service thus mandates goals for nursing practice. Moreover, there are background values, such as the commitment to individual autonomy or to beneficence, which inform the practice of nursing. As Donaldson and Crowley put the point:

> *"Ethical and moral values inherent in clinical practice have profoundly influenced the perspective and value orientation of the discipline. Thus, nursing has traditionally valued humanitarian service. But in addition, the self-respect and self-determination of clients are to be preserved. The goal of nursing service is to foster self-caring behavior that leads to individual health and well-being."* (Donaldson & Crowley, 1978, p. 117)

There are, then, values embedded in professional practice, and these values have a dynamic relationship to the society and institutions in which professional nurses work. These values, in turn, influence the discipline:

> *"These values and goals, which are intrinsic to professional practice, have shaped the value orientation of the discipline. As a result of this value orientation, knowledge of the basis of human choices and of methods for fostering individual independence are sought, rather than knowledge of interventions that control and directly manipulate the person per se into a societally determined state of health."* (Donaldson & Crowley, 1978, p. 117)

Citing Johnson (1974), Donaldson and Crowley note that the values implicit in the clinical practice of nursing influence "the decisions about what to study and what questions to ask" (Donaldson & Crowley, 1978, p. 117).

The picture that emerges of the relationship between disciplinary knowledge and the value orientation of the professional practice is like a feedback loop. There is a dynamic relationship between the values intrinsic to the profession and the larger society that gives nursing its mandate. The values intrinsic to the profession determine the topics, general themes, or fundamental questions of the discipline. The science of nursing then takes up these topics, themes, and questions, and uses scientific methods to develop and test theories. These empirical theories are then the substance of the discipline, the fundamental knowledge that informs nursing practice. The discipline of nursing thus provides the intellectual expertise that grounds the claim to professional status. As the discipline develops, and the knowledge base expands, the areas of nursing expertise will change. As nursing expertise grows, the social mandate for nursing can and should be modified. Changes in nursing roles might modify some of the values intrinsic to practice, beginning the process all over again.

The Johnson–Donaldson–Crowley model relates the values of the profession to disciplinary knowledge by treating the values as guides for the science. The professional values focus attention on certain problems, themes, or questions. To get a critical grip on this model, there are two kinds of question we need to ask. First, there is a cluster of epistemological questions. Does this way of relating nursing values to nursing science keep nursing science "value-free"? Does it undermine, or does it preserve, the objectivity of nursing science? Second, any good model of how nursing values relate to nursing science must make sense of the way nursing practice, research, and theory development *actually* work. So, of any such model, we need to ask whether it is an adequate account of the discipline and professional practice of nursing as they work on the ground, so to speak. Of course, the two kinds of question work together. It could be that "on the ground" nursing research and practice is not epistemically sound. This would be a reason to change the practice. On the other hand, it might be that some philosophical ways of understanding epistemology are a better fit for practice, and this is at least a prima facie reason to prefer some philosophical accounts.

Constitutive and contextual values

Research in the philosophy of science over the past 30 years has developed some conceptual tools that will help us sharpen the questions about how professional values are related to nursing science. As with so many philosophical tools, this one takes the form of a series of distinctions. With these distinctions in hand, we will be able to map the conceptual territory, and thereby get a clearer sense of what commitments are required by various philosophical positions.

In the 1980s and 1990s, philosophers of science began to invoke a distinction between "constitutive" and "contextual" values (McMullin, 1983; Longino, 1990). This is not a distinction between kinds of value, but a distinction between the ways a value-judgment might influence an activity. That is, it is a distinction in kinds of function or role for values. A value-judgment has a constitutive role when it is intrinsic to, or necessary for, an activity. For example, the goal of winning is intrinsic to a game of checkers; the value of an education is intrinsic to teaching. When a value has a constitutive role in an activity, the activity requires commitment to the value. We might say that it is presupposed in the sense that, without it, the activity could not proceed in its ordinary form. Those who place no value on winning are not playing checkers, at least not in a serious way. Or again, it is a poor teacher who places no value on the students' education. In the absence of commitment to the constitutive values, the actors are just going through the motions.

Contextual values, on the other hand, are not necessary for, or required by, the activity. Participants may hold such values or not, but in either case, they are participating in a full-blooded way. Both checkers and teaching can be pursued professionally. The money earned is valuable to the participants, but neither teaching nor playing checkers requires payment. Unpaid teaching and amateur checkers are not ersatz forms of teaching or checkers. Notice that contextual values may influence or shape the activity. Professionalizing a game can force changes in rules or strategy. There are, for example, "TV time-outs" in professional basketball. These are forced by commercial breaks, but they give the players a chance to catch their breath and discuss strategy, thus making televised games different from untelevised games. In spite of their influence, such values remain contextual because commitment to them is not required or presupposed by the activity. A professional basketball player might give all of his earnings to charity, and he would be no less of a basketball player.

Applied to science, the constitutive/contextual distinction helps show how science can be put in service of, and even influenced by, public policy without being tainted by politics. Public policy and social values are part of the context within which science operates. Political decisions and social values determine the priorities for funding scientific research. Ethical decisions (sometimes expressed institutionally in the form of ethics review boards) influence choice of method and study populations. These contextual values shape the science. They influence the topics investigated and the methods of investigation. However, once the topics and methods are chosen, science proceeds independently of the social values or political priorities. As scientists in many oppressive political regimes have learned, good science can take place in an environment where the scope of research is severely constrained. One way for science to be value-free, then, is for there to be no constitutive values in science. Johnson's model, as developed by Beckstrand, Carper, Donaldson and Crowley, makes science value-free in this sense. Carper and Beckstrand express a conception of science (empirics) that is value-free in the sense that there are no constitutive values. All value-commitments are contained within the ethical pattern of knowing. On the Johnson model, professional values in nursing set the topics, themes, and questions for the science of nursing. In this way, they shape nursing science, but nursing science does not need to incorporate professional values in any deep way. If professional values are merely contextual, the content of nursing science is value-free.

Constitutive values in science: Kuhn's argument

As we saw in the previous chapter, Dickoff and James wanted to include the goals of nursing within the scope of situation-producing theory. This would make professional values constitutive of nursing inquiry. We also saw that there were a number of ways in which nursing science might need to incorporate values, from Yeo's discussion of "managing stimuli" to White's sociopolitical knowing. Is there any way to understand science as having *constitutive* values that maintain its epistemic respectability?

Thomas Kuhn provided one argument showing that scientific practice may require value-judgments. In "Objectivity, value judgment, and theory choice," Kuhn argued that value-commitments were an ineliminable part of theory development and testing (Kuhn, 1977). A central business of science is to develop theories and to replace inadequate theories with better ones. Theories are judged on the basis of accuracy, consistency, scope, simplicity, and so on. Clearly, more accurate theories are preferable to less accurate ones. Kuhn argued that these criteria for theory choice functioned as values. Notice that these are criteria for theory choice, that is, they are criteria for judging that one theory is better than another. Kuhn argued that, historically, scientists have disagreed about which of the criteria is more important.

As an example of Kuhn's thesis, consider the dispute between two historical astronomers, Ptolemy and Copernicus, about the solar system. Retrograde motion is one of the striking phenomena of astronomy. Each night, the planet Mars (for example) will appear a little to the east of where it appeared the night before. However, after several weeks, the planet seems to reverse its course and moves back to the west. Then it reverses again and continues east. Over a number of weeks, the planet seems to move in great loop through the sky. Ancient astronomers thought that the sun, stars, and planets revolved around the earth. The sun and moon seem to have natural, circular paths. The retrograde motion of Mars and the other planets was a challenge to explain.

Ptolemy (circa 85–165 C.E.) explained retrograde motion by postulating that the planets actually move in a looping orbit. He created a geometric representation of the motion that accurately predicted where the planets would appear in the night sky. Copernicus (1473–1543 C.E.) put the sun at the center of the solar system. He postulated that the planets moved on simple circular paths around the sun. He explained retrograde motion as an illusion. The Earth has a shorter path around the sun. As it catches up and passes Mars, Mars seems to stop and move backwards, just as a car seems to move backwards as it is passed on the highway.

The Copernican model of the solar system made predictions about where the planets would be found in the night sky, but interestingly, it was *less accurate* than the Ptolemaic model. Nonetheless, Galileo and other scientists preferred Copernicus' model because it was simpler and more consistent with their theories of motion. Kuhn argued that it was not irrational for a Ptolemaic astronomer to reject Copernicus' model of the solar system. After all, it was less accurate. Similarly, Copernicans could reject the Ptolemaic model on the grounds that it was unnecessarily complicated. The decision to accept one theory rather than another, Kuhn concluded, depends in part[1] on the decision to prioritize accuracy over simplicity (or vice versa). Accuracy, simplicity, consistency, etc., thus function as values that guide theory choice.

Epistemic and moral/political values

Deciding among rival theories is, arguably, a central part of scientific practice. Kuhn argued that value-judgments are a necessary part of theory choice. They are, therefore, constitutive of scientific inquiry. Once we recognize these criteria as values that play a role in science, it is apparent that science is shot through with such values. Many scientific activities require judgments that one result, method, or theory is better than another. It is *good* for lab assistants to clean the equipment, for epidemiological samples to be representative, and for interviews to be honest. These are also value-judgments, and it is quite clear that science could not proceed without them. This is an important, but limited, conclusion. It is important because it shows that science is not a matter of reading truths from the book of nature. Evaluative judgment is a crucial part of the process. At the same time, the values seem benign; accuracy and simplicity may be values, but they are not moral values such as equality and autonomy. It is not too troubling to find that values such as accuracy or parsimony are constitutive of science.

To get a better fix on the problems at hand, then, we might distinguish *epistemic* values from political or moral values. Accuracy and simplicity are epistemic values in the sense that they are criteria that guide us when our goal is a true description of our world. Given that we want to know the truth, accurate, simple, and consistent theories are good guides. Moral and political values, on the other hand, seem more problematic when they appear in scientific reasoning. The fact that a theory is judged to be politically expedient is a very poor reason to think that it accurately depicts the world.

Models of value-laden inquiry

The two distinctions—constitutive versus contextual, epistemic versus moral/political—cut across one another, creating four possibilities for values in scientific inquiry:

1. Constitutive epistemic	2. Contextual epistemic
3. Constitutive moral/political	4. Contextual moral/political

Beckstrand and Carper separated ethics and empirics into distinct patterns. They held that science is value-free, but that it occurred in the context of professional

---

[1] Historically speaking, of course, the story is much more complicated.

values. Therefore, using this rubric, we might portray their view as saying that there are no constitutive values in nursing science. That is, there is nothing in cells (1) and (3). All values that properly influence science—whether epistemic or moral/political—are contextual:

1. Constitutive epistemic	2. Contextual epistemic
3. Constitutive moral/political	4. Contextual moral/political

Kuhn's argument (above) challenges this strict separation. Most philosophers of science today will agree that there are values that fit into cell (1). This admission does not disrupt Donaldson and Crowley's explanation of how professional values influence the discipline. Nursing science might require constitutive, epistemic values, but the moral and political values of the profession remain contextual. In the diagram, there would be values in cell (1), but not in (3):

1. Constitutive epistemic	2. Contextual epistemic
3. Constitutive moral/political	4. Contextual moral/political

This position would exclude the most troublesome values (moral or political values) from a constitutive role in science. But because only epistemic values are constitutive, the values enhance objectivity rather than detract from it. Understanding nursing science in these terms would make it value-laden, yet at the same time preserve a traditional conception of scientific objectivity.

Value-laden concepts in nursing inquiry

The discussion of how professional values influence nursing science in Chapter 4 challenges the moderate thesis just articulated. Yeo argued that terms like "managing stimuli" were value-laden. Since the implicit values are moral, this argument would show that there were constitutive moral values in nursing science (cell 3, above). But how widespread are such value-laden concepts in nursing? To answer this question, perhaps it is best to start with the most fundamental notions.

Donaldson and Crowley's three themes are widely recognized as the orienting ideas of nursing inquiry (Donaldson & Crowley, 1978, p. 113 italics added):

1. Concern with principles and laws that govern the life processes, *well-being*, and *optimum functioning* of human beings.
2. Concern with the patterning of human behavior in interaction with the environment in *critical* life situations.
3. Concern with the processes by which *positive changes* in *health* status are affected.

Each of the italicized terms is arguably value-laden. The most obvious are "well-being" and "positive changes." Both presuppose that some states of health are better than others, and we ought to aim at achieving and maintaining them. "Critical life situations" is a bit more subtle. "Critical" is, after all, used as a technical term for patients who are in danger of dying. In a nursing context, however, the term cannot be so restricted. The critical life situations with which nurses are concerned are not limited to cardiac arrest or kidney failure. Death of a spouse, diagnosis of a fatal condition, or loss of ability are among the profound human experiences that count as critical life situations for nursing. These are critical because they have consequences for our happiness and for the way we conduct our lives. "Critical life situations" is therefore a value-laden concept.

The master concept, of course, is *health*, and is not news to nurses that this concept is value-laden. It is hard to disagree with Sally Thorne and her colleagues that "a majority of nursing theorists have conceptualized health as a normative state and/or process" (Thorne *et al.*, 1998, p. 1261). In philosophy, the claim has been more controversial. Some, most notably Christopher Boorse (1977, 1981, 1997), have tried to articulate a concept of health that is descriptive and value-free. For Boorse, the value-free sense of "health" is the opposite of disease. A disease, according to Boorse's analysis, is a deviation from the normal function of the organism. Following this analysis, "optimum functioning" would be characterized in terms of the statistical and functional norms of the human species, in the way that normal vision is defined as 20/20. Philosophers have criticized Boorse's arguments, arguing that health is value-laden in one way or another (Margolis, 1976; Culver & Gert, 1982; Nordenfelt, 1987; Seedhouse, 2001).

This philosophical controversy has little grip in the nursing context. The professional responsibilities of nurses cannot be limited to the optimum functioning of the organism. An 80-year-old and a 30-year-old may have the same dysfunction. But from a nursing standpoint, these patients require very different responses. The potentialities, well-being, and preferences of the patient must be taken into account when the nurse creates her care plan.[2] The debate in nursing is not whether health (and related concepts such as well-being or quality of life) is value-free, but whether the values can be disentangled from the nurse's response to the whole person (Ellis, 1982; Mitchell & Cody, 1992; Cody, 1995; Thorne *et al.*, 1998).

As a focus for disciplinary inquiry in nursing, then, health is a value-laden concept. Moreover, the values that inform the concept of health are not epistemic values. While health is not commonly part of ethical theories, it is clearly a human good. It is part of what we consider human flourishing, and all humans try to maintain their health or recover it when lost. In this broad sense, health is a moral concept. Recognizing that the concept of health is normative, however, does not entail that it is *entirely* normative. Health is an example of a "thick" moral concept. Bernard Williams distinguished between thick and thin moral concepts, and the difference is helpful here (Williams, 1985, p. 140). In the moral theories of philosophy, the concepts discussed have minimal descriptive content. Moral theory aims to

---

[2] In Boorse's terms, nurses respond to the patient's illness. Since illness is a value-laden notion, the concept of health in nursing is value-laden, on Boorse's analysis. Nordenfelt has argued that the same is true of the physician (2007, p. 8).

understand what is morally right (good, just, virtuous, etc.) in a way that transcends differences among people or their situations. In this sense, philosophical concepts in ethics are very "thin." Many of the moral concepts we use every day, however, have descriptive content. The differences among the concepts of rape, incest, sexual abuse, and sexual harassment are differences in the descriptive or factual commitments that each concept involves. In other words, the difference between a case of rape and a case of sexual abuse is found in the facts of the case, not in the moral wrongness of the action. Health, disease, and illness are also thick moral concepts. They have both moral and descriptive elements to their meaning.

Conclusion: constitutive moral and political values in nursing inquiry

If the arguments of the foregoing section are sound, then some *constitutive* values of nursing inquiry are not merely *epistemic*. (In other words, all of the cells of the diagrams above have contents.) It follows that Carper's segregation of ethical and empiric patterns of knowing is a profound misrepresentation of nursing knowledge. The focal topics of nursing inquiry cannot and should not be understood in purely descriptive, factual terms. The key concepts have moral (or political) dimensions that could not be eliminated. White's sociopolitical pattern integrated empirical knowledge and political commitment, and it is supported by the foregoing considerations. However, while this conclusion vindicates sociopolitical knowing in nursing, it also shows why treating it as a fifth pattern would be mistaken. As a fifth pattern, it would preserve the (value-free) empirics and (valued-laden) ethics patterns. The lesson to be drawn from the foregoing reflections is that the distinction among the patterns cannot be maintained. The empiric pattern is already sociopolitical.

These arguments also have ramifications for the Johnson–Donaldson–Crowley model of how professional values influence nursing science. As we have seen, this model presupposes that nursing science is (or should be) value-free. Professional values play only a contextual role, indirectly influencing nursing science by motivating the topics. The arguments above show that the discipline of nursing has constitutive, moral, or political values built into the topics of inquiry. This implies that the profession and the discipline are more intimately related than the Johnson–Donaldson–Crowley model suggests.

Standpoint epistemology and nursing knowledge

In the previous chapter, we saw how moral and political values associated with the profession are built into the content of some of the key concepts of the discipline. This shows that moral and political values are not always harmful. An inquiry can have constitutive moral values without undermining its status as a legitimate scientific enterprise. Feminist philosophers of science have developed a stronger position, arguing that under the right conditions politically informed inquiry can make science better. This kind of view, generally known as "standpoint epistemology," looks to the social position of the investigator for values that will inform the inquiry. The moral and political values important to nursing knowledge have their grounds in the roles of professional nurses. What can standpoint epistemology tell us about the relation between nursing values and nursing knowledge?

Social role and epistemic privilege

According to standpoint theorists,[1] some social roles (standpoints) can generate more accurate knowledge of particular domains than others. The idea has its roots in Marx's analysis of ideology, but in recent work by feminists has freed it from Marx's idiosyncrasies. Many social theorists have held that social relationships are ultimately determined by what people do. Marx[2] called the human activities at the foundation of society "material practices." These are concrete interactions among people, and between humans and their environment: barter, planting crops, or paying wages to laborers. Power is not always (perhaps never) equal in a society, and this is manifested in the practical ways in which people relate to each other. Within

---

[1] For classic papers in feminist standpoint theory, see (Harding, 2003).
[2] This presentation of Marxist standpoint epistemology is largely based on Nancy Hartsock (1983).

a capitalist society, Marx thought, there is a dominant, ruling class and a working class. The ruling class determines many of the material practices that constitute the very social relations that keep them in power. For example, by paying wages for some kinds of work and not others, the dominant class simultaneously creates and marginalizes different ways of life. The working class' cooperation in the system is necessary, for they provide the labor that drives capitalism.

While social relationships are constituted by material practices, and thus by what people do, participants do not always have an accurate understanding of their own society. Marx claimed that a distorted view of social relationships is an important part of what keeps the ruling class in power. "Ideology" is the Marxist term for the distorted view held by the dominant class. For example, according to Marx, the factory owner needs to see his bargaining with the workers as a process of free and open exchange. This permits the owner to maintain the idea that his labor arrangements are fair and just. The social reality might be quite different: if the laborer has no way to feed his family other than working at the factory, it is not exactly a free and open exchange.

Since the factory owner has power over the arrangements, he creates the material practices that constitute the real social relationship. Hence, while his view is distorted, it is not utterly mistaken. The worker, on the other hand, is in a position to understand more about the relationship between himself and the factory owner. He feels the injustices of the bargain for wages because he knows he is making a forced choice. Yet, as a participant in the relationship created (in large part) by the owner, he can understand it from the factory owner's perspective too. The worker—and, Marx argued, the working class in general—is thus in a position to see social relationships *both* from the perspective of the ruling class *and* the perspective of the laborers who make the system work. Of course, not every member of the working class will have an accurate understanding of the social structure. The ideology of the ruling class distorts the working class viewpoint as well as their own. The standpoint of the working class requires struggle, in particular, political struggle. The political goals of Marxism thus require epistemic change as well as political change.

Feminist appropriation of standpoint epistemology

Feminist theorists (e.g., Hartsock, 1983) and social scientists (e.g., Smith, 1974) noticed the obvious parallels between gender and class relationships. Insofar as men hold power in a society, they control the material practices that constitute social relations. Masculine dominance, however, is not strictly economic. Indeed, one of the objections that feminists had to Marxism is that women's work in the home was invisible to standard models of economic exchange. Nonetheless, women's work makes the male roles possible in much the same way as Marx saw workers supporting the capitalist system. Women are in a position to understand both the partial, male perspective and understand what makes that perspective possible. Thus, women are in a position to achieve a more adequate understanding of society, especially the ways in which society is structured by gender. And again, this more adequate understanding requires both political change and empirical inquiry.

Feminist scholars were thus able to generalize the Marxian idea that the working class was in a privileged epistemic position with respect to social relationships. Social structures (whether in the domestic sphere or outside of it) are such that persons who occupy some social positions are unable to get a clear understanding of the society in which they live. A perspective is privileged when one can see things that the other perspective cannot see *and* understand why the other cannot see it. Women, the working class, and (in the West) people of color[3] are in such a position. Since the knower exists within the very social structures that distort understanding, the knowledge made possible by an epistemic standpoint is not immediate. The achievement of the knowledge available to a standpoint takes scientific inquiry and a political commitment to making the social structures more just. This is the precise sense in which some standpoints (in particular, those of women, people of color, and the proletariat) are epistemically privileged.

Early versions of feminist standpoint epistemology faced some important challenges. First, feminists were in the apparently paradoxical position of wanting to argue against male-biased science, yet in favor of science informed by feminist values. This made some critics think that feminist science was little more than the demand that science supports feminist values (Antony, 1993; Haack, 1993; Hekman, 1997). It was epistemologically no better off than the androcentric science it sought to criticize. In responding to these criticisms, feminist philosophers have improved our understanding of how values figure in scientific research (Longino, 1990; Harding, 1991; Anderson, 1995; Wylie, 2002). Not all values undermine objectivity, and objectivity can be improved when the certain values play the right roles. Contemporary standpoint epistemology arguably shows how feminist political goals can be part of an empirically robust and realistic philosophy of science.

Another problem for early versions of standpoint epistemology was that they "essentialized" gender, race, and class. Standpoint epistemology argues that only from oppressed positions can one explain why the dominant group has a distorted understanding of social relationships. In Marxian theory, this explanation relied on the mechanisms of ideology and class consciousness. Early feminist writing on standpoint epistemology replaced this with a psychodynamic account of male and female development (so-called "object-relations theory" cf. Chodorow, 1978; Fox Keller, 1978). However, both sorts of explanation have the unfortunate effect of making certain attributes of the group essential. In the same period where feminist standpoint theory was being developed, other feminist theorists were arguing that we

---

[3] The analysis has been applied to race by Collins (2000). Race is a crucial dimension of analysis for contemporary standpoint epistemology. It has been left out here for the sake of a simpler presentation of the main ideas. Historically, nursing has been a profession available to oppressed or marginalized people of color. Therefore, a full understanding of the nursing standpoint will require understanding the way in which race intersects the other analytical categories. These include not only race, gender, and class, but also, as will be argued below, the division of labor in health care.

should reject essentializing depictions of women. Gender, they argued, is a social construction; gender attributes have a history, and that history is laden with problematic political values. Insofar as standpoint epistemology assumed that there was a unitary and necessary position of "woman" or "worker," it was at odds with other feminist commitments.

Generalizing standpoints

Standpoint epistemologists of the 1990s began to think that the strong commitments of class consciousness or object-relations theory were unnecessary. A commitment to different social roles for men and women is sufficient to generate the epistemological difference required by standpoint epistemology. This permitted standpoint epistemology to embrace the diversity of women's roles, experiences, and ways of being (Harding, 1991). On this view, an epistemically privileged standpoint exists whenever a pair of social roles satisfies the following conditions:

1.   One role is oppressed[4] relative to another, dominant role.
2.   The relationship between the roles is structured by the needs and interests of the dominant role.
3.   The practices of the subordinate role make the activities of the dominant role possible, and these activities are largely invisible to the dominant group.
4.   In order to fulfill their role, those who occupy the subordinate role need to understand some domain from both the perspective of the dominant role and from their own perspective.

When the members of an oppressed group meet these four conditions, and when they are committed to valorizing or ameliorating their condition, it will be possible for them to reach a clearer and more adequate understanding of the social situation. This requires inquiry that begins from the lives of the oppressed or marginalized group. It must recognize their challenges as real problems to be solved, and it must be politically committed to solving them. Moreover, since the subordinate group participates in a relationship structured by the dominant group, they will be in a position to understand both the dominant "ideology" and their own experience of how that dominant group is supported and its dominance maintained. Under the right conditions, then, incorporating political commitments into empirical inquiry produces a clearer, less distorted view of some domain. Such value-laden inquiry is arguably *more* objective in such circumstances than its (purportedly) value-free counterparts, a point sometimes expressed with the phrase "strong objectivity" (cf. Harding, 1995).

   Contemporary health care is a mosaic of roles that divide labor as well as knowledge. Can the standpoint analysis be extended to the relationship between doctors

---

[4] "Oppression" is a blanket term that covers a number of different conditions. The oppression need not take the form of economic injustice; the subordinate group may be marginalized or silenced in other ways (Young, 1988).

and nurses? The history of nursing provides the first hint. When Florence Nightingale secularized and professionalized the role of the nurse, she established the domain of nursing expertise. This domain was a necessary part of patient care, and it was distinct from the physician's domain of diagnosis and treatment. Nightingale's division of labor in health care was self-consciously constructed in parallel with Victorian gender roles. The domain of expertise allocated to nurses was already the domain of governesses and mothers. Nightingale understood herself to be valorizing and professionalizing the woman's role in (upper and middle class) Victorian society. For example, in the conclusion to *Notes on Nursing* she considers the objection that her work of educating women as nurses will lead to "amateur physicking." She responds that

> "*to cultivate in things pertaining to health observation and experience in women who are mothers, governesses or nurses, is just the way to do away with amateur physicking, and if the doctors did not know it, to make the nurses obedient to them,—helps to them instead of hindrances.*" (Nightingale, [1860] 1969, p. 130)

Nightingale thus built the power asymmetry between men and women into the relation between doctors and nurses. If standpoint epistemology is right, then such asymmetries of power can indeed produce powerful asymmetries of knowledge. Does the position of a nurse within the health care hierarchy provide a kind of epistemic privilege?

Knowledge and the division of labor in health care

The foregoing section identified four conditions that need to be satisfied if a social role is to constitute an epistemic standpoint. Substantial evidence that nursing satisfies these four conditions can be found in Maureen Coombs's *Power and Conflict between Doctors and Nurses* (2004). Coombs's study was an ethnography of three British intensive care units. These were adult care facilities, housing between 10 and 18 beds, and serving between 500 and 1500 patients per year. The primary focus of her research was "the way that knowledge and roles are used within the decision-making process in the delivery of health care" (Coombs, 2004, p. xv). To uncover these processes, Coombs conducted interviews and observed ward rounds. Rounds are crucial sites for understanding how power and knowledge interact. Coombs found that both physicians and nurses used the biomedical model of health and the associated knowledge of physiological systems in their response to the patient. An excerpt from her field notes shows how biomedical knowledge permeated their conversations:

> "DOCTOR: *So how's it going here?* NURSE: *Well, let's see, resp [respiratory] wise we're fully ventilated and on high FIO$_2$. She's still desaturating on turning, so we're hyper-oxygenating her. Cardiovascular, well she's on Norad with mean arterial pressures of 70. We're volume loading her, and her acidosis is worsening. What parameters are we*

working towards? I'm sure she's overloaded. Anyhow, her urine was 20 mls this hour." (Coombs, 2004, p. 64)

This sort of information is crucial to decision-making in contemporary health care. It is not surprising that both physicians and nurses were fluent and comfortable with the language of chemistry, pharmacology, and physiology. Coombs documents that, in ward rounds, the biomedical model permeated the discussion, and it was the primary ground for decisions about patient treatment.

Both physicians and nurses recognized that nursing expertise was distinct from a physician's expertise. As one physician in Coombs's study put it: "There are certain areas in the ward round that I bequeath to nursing—the choice of beds, those clinically superficial areas—bowel care, skin care, mouth care, wound care" (Coombs, 2004, p. 65). In addition to these well-known sites of nursing care, Coombs documented other areas of recognized nursing expertise. The first concerned the family and social situation of the patient. Nurses were the primary liaison between the family and the medical world of the hospital. Since they understood the technical aspects of care, they could explain procedures and help the family anticipate outcomes. Where the patient was unconscious, their relationship with the family helped provide relevant information about the patient. Discussion of the patient's family was a routine part of patient handover among nurses. The nursing documentation included the patient's social relationships and any information shared with the family (Coombs, 2004, p. 71).

A further area of nursing expertise arose from the nurse's continuous presence with the patient. The three units studied by Coombs aimed for a one-to-one patient-to-nurse ratio. As a result, nurses had detailed knowledge of how the patients were responding to treatment, to sedation, and to analgesia. They knew whether the patient had a rough night, or would get uncomfortable as levels of sedation were reduced. Finally, nursing expertise included the patient's physical environment and its management. Some of this knowledge concerned the hospital organization and systems: requisition of supplies, implementation of safety and incident policies, and personnel management. An important aspect of this environmental knowledge was the nurses' ability to manipulate the equipment that is a necessary part of intensive care. Coombs documented that nurses, not physicians, had the ability to use the equipment and the responsibility to be sure that it was working properly. It is interesting that the subjects of Coombs's study did not recognize this area of expertise as a kind of knowledge:

"When I discussed this knowledge with medical and nursing staff, it became clear that skills required, for example, to prime an infusion set to deliver medication or manage a staff budget, were just accepted as 'part of the job'. Such activities were not seen as a source of knowledge." (Coombs, 2004, p. 79)

Some abilities that are a necessary part of nursing were thus invisible to both nurses and physicians. Coombs suggests that this is because the knowledge is practical, implicit, or tacit. As is so often the case with abilities, the fact that one knows how to do something does not rise to consciousness until there is a failure or breakdown.

All of the areas of knowledge, both shared and unique, were important to the decisions made about patient treatment. However, physicians—and to some extent nurses too—disvalued the nursing expertise over the shared biomedical knowledge. The areas "bequeathed" to nursing were "clinically superficial." Nursing expertise seemed routinely dismissed in Coombs's interviews with physicians:

> *"I mean the nurses come on at 8, they come into the office with their coffee for 'handover' and for allocation—God only knows what they talk about—it's not a handover, it's a chat. They then come out and get a second handover from the patient's nurse, about nursey things, about relatives, not medical things."* (Coombs, 2004, p. 73)

Coombs's observation of ward rounds documented that the domains of nursing knowledge were recognized only as peripheral issues. Biomedical issues constituted the bulk of the discussion in ward rounds. Issues about relatives, continuity of treatment, patient comfort, and so on tended to be tagged on at the end, if mentioned at all. Occasionally, the team would turn to the nurse for a report, but the nurses felt they had to be very assertive if their concerns were to be heard (Coombs, 2004, p. 101ff).

Coombs's study thus found both power and knowledge differentials between doctors and nurses. Nurses had recognized expertise in several areas: an up-close knowledge of how the patient was responding to treatment, the performance of bodily functions that are essential to life and health but not the focus of treatment, the management of the patient's physical environment, and the patient's social relationships. In addition, nurses were conversant with contemporary biomedicine and were able to communicate with the physicians in these terms. The power differential between physicians and nurses was replicated in the relationship between their respective areas of expertise. The physician's knowledge was treated as the more important form, and the areas of nursing expertise were marginalized. It is interesting that, in spite of the frustration nurses sometimes felt, both physicians and nurses treated the nursing expertise as secondary to the physician's knowledge.

Nursing knowledge and nursing roles

It is not difficult to see the social roles of nurses as satisfying the four criteria for an epistemically privileged standpoint. First, the role of the nurse in health care is oppressed and marginalized as compared with the role of the physician. For centuries, physicians have dominated the practice of medicine. Even though the discipline of nursing has worked hard to get recognition for the contributions of nurses, they participate in a system where their role is largely determined by the needs of physicians. In Coombs's study, physicians and nurses regarded the physicians as the primary decision-makers, and their discourse dominated the rounds. The nurses' expertise was treated as a "superficial" addition. Second, the relationship between physicians and nurses is largely structured by the needs of physicians. Since Nightingale's time, the boundaries of potential nursing concern have been set by the limits of physician interest. The sites of nursing care (hygiene, wound care, monitoring, regulation of medication, interaction with hospital systems, and so on) are all determined by the needs of the patient, *given* the prescribed treatment regime. Even as they have gained autonomy within the health care system, nurses' responsibilities have been harnessed to the physicians' treatment regimen.

Third, while the nursing role is necessary for the physicians, nursing work is largely invisible. Without the nursing care in all of its aspects, the treatment regimen could not be successful. This is striking in intensive care wards, but no less true in other circumstances. It is not that physicians do not know what nurses do. Rather, as the physicians' remarks in Coombs's study show, they do not appreciate the ways in which nursing work makes their treatment possible. To regard nursing as concerned with things that are "clinically superficial" is to betray a deep misunderstanding. By tending to bodily needs, by providing care for pain or insomnia, or by counseling and educating, nursing creates an environment within which the physician's treatment can be effective.

Finally, nurses need to understand the patient's health from both the physician's perspective and their own. Knowing the patient in the physician's terms is necessary for their supporting role. Coombs's study documented how the nurses were fluent in the language of biomedicine, and they mobilized the same knowledge as the physicians. They used this to manage the patient directly (monitoring blood chemistry, etc.), and to anticipate the physician's concerns (aiming for parameters). The nurse's understanding cannot be limited to the knowledge shared with physicians because the health needs to which she responds are more comprehensive. In a literal sense, nurses know what happens to the patient after the physician has left the room.

The crucial, final ingredient of a standpoint epistemology is the political commitment to develop the knowledge available to those who occupy the marginalized social role. The knowledge available to a standpoint is not automatic; it requires political commitment and empirical work. This is where the nursing role differs from the typical loci of standpoint analysis. For the standpoints of class, gender, and race, the political commitment is to social justice. In nursing, the commitment is to the values at the core of nursing practice, including the patient's autonomy and well-being, as well as to the valorization of the nursing role itself. These values motivate the empirical project of embedding the view of human health as disease and dysfunction into a larger picture that includes the psychological, social, and personal elements of health. This attempt to synthesize physiology, pharmacology, pathology, psychology, and sociology, and to focus them on the patient and the patient's experience, is the science of nursing. This highlights a further difference between the nursing standpoint and class, gender, or racial standpoints. While the traditional standpoints have the potential to provide a less distorted view of social relationships, the nursing standpoint can provide a less distorted view of human health.

Conclusion: nursing knowledge as an epistemic standpoint

There are deeply entrenched and widespread constitutive values in the disciplinary knowledge base of nursing. The Johnson–Donaldson–Crowley model used the professional values of nursing to direct the central topics of the discipline. This chapter has argued that these values can play an even more important role in nursing knowledge. Standpoint epistemology relies on the idea that moral or political values can be constitutive to scientific inquiry. Given a commitment to the central values of nursing, the knowledge that nurses have of human health in virtue of the special role they play in health care can be uncovered. Nursing knowledge would therefore be an outgrowth of the nursing standpoint.

The nursing standpoint

Top-down and bottom-up views of nursing

In the late 1970s, a consensus formed about the character of the nursing discipline (cf. Chapter 2). It defined the field of nursing as an inquiry into a specific set of topics (Donaldson and Crowley's three themes, Fawcett's metaparadigm). These themes were identified by the core values of the profession and its social mandate. The second point of consensus was that nursing science is hierarchically organized. Grand theory provides the most abstract and general investigation into the unifying themes and concepts of nursing. Mid-range theory gives specific, empirical content to the generalizations of grand theory. Theories developed at this level can then be applied to nursing practice through the development of specific interventions. The discipline of nursing thus "governs" the profession by providing both directives for practice and the content of nursing expertise. Because the scope of nursing expertise should determine the scope of nursing practice, on this view, the proper boundaries of the nursing profession are finally set by the discipline. It is, in a sense, a top-down view of the unity of nursing.

If nursing knowledge is understood as an epistemic standpoint—the nursing standpoint—then a radically different philosophical picture emerges. Fundamentally, the practice and the discipline of nursing are in an intimate and dynamic relationship. The slogan of feminist standpoint epistemology is that research should start "from the perspectives of women's lives" (Harding, 1991, p. 249). The slogan of a nursing standpoint would be that research should start from the perspectives of *nurses'* lives. This means that the problems and questions of nursing research must, in the first instance, be problems and questions that arise from nursing practice. In their daily work, nurses in hospitals, clinics, schools, homes, and public health institutions encounter and solve problems. All of these require knowledge, and the nurses' expertise lies in their ability to handle all of the problems that are thrown at them. Some of this expertise is know-how gained through persistence and hard work; some of it is gained through training and education. The enterprise of nursing science is to develop, refine, and expand the intellectual expertise of professional nurses.

Saying that the problems and questions of nursing research must arise from nursing practice has two implications. First, some knowledge is embedded in practice, and as nurse scholars from Orlando to Benner have argued, one function of nursing research is to unearth this knowledge, refine it, test it, and communicate it to others. Second, there is the mobilization of theoretical knowledge. Some of this knowledge has been developed by nurse researchers, but it also comes from other sources. Nurse education draws on the biomedical sciences, psychology, sociology, and education, not to mention the humanities. All of this knowledge is part of nursing expertise insofar as it helps solve the difficulties with which the nurse is faced. The second implication of the slogan that research should start from the perspectives of *nurses'* lives, then, is that nursing scholarship must develop theories that speak to the needs of practitioners.

On the consensus view of the nursing discipline, Donaldson and Crowley's three themes and Fawcett's four concepts of the metaparadigm give the discipline its distinctive character. It is a top-down model of disciplinary unity. According to it, inquiry counts as nursing research when it employs these concepts and investigates those topics. On the standpoint view, the discipline of nursing gets its unity from the bottom up. Professional values do not isolate a set of abstract topics; they identify particular nursing problems to be solved. Research and theory development are appropriately part of the nursing discipline when they respond to nursing problems. The response need not be immediate. The nursing standpoint does not require all research to focus on interventions and outcomes. Most difficult problems can only be fully resolved by deep understanding. This requires theory. From the nursing standpoint, it does not matter whether the theory was developed entirely by nurse researchers or whether it is borrowed, whole or in part, from other sciences. A theory is appropriate for the nursing discipline when it addresses nursing problems. Its provenance has little interest. The nursing standpoint thus permits a view of interdisciplinary research similar to that found in other disciplines where complex, multidimensional phenomena are studied. Scholars in social psychology or environmental health adopt and develop theories that originated in a wide variety of disciplines, and their research is stronger for it. According to the standpoint view, nursing should do so too.

Values in the nursing standpoint

The professional values of nursing mediate the relationship between theory and practice, and they do so in several ways. What nurses take to be good or bad for the client determine what problems need to be solved. And the values involved, when understood in their full, rich context, are distinctive of the nursing enterprise. For example, valuing patient autonomy is common to the twenty-first century health professions. But for nurses, autonomy means more than informed consent and the right to refuse treatment. Nursing tries to develop and support the autonomy of patients. Patients are made better decision-makers through nurse education, and better at self-care through nursing interventions. That a patient cannot feed him- or herself is a problem for nursing because of the value nurses place on enhancing personal autonomy. Notice that the values do not pick out abstract topics; they make very specific needs salient. The knowledge used to resolve the problems is made valuable in the same stroke. The required knowledge might be a specific, nurse-designed intervention, or it might be drawn from more general theories in psychology, sociology, or physiology. Starting inquiry from nurses' lives, then, requires that nurse researchers recognize the problems of practice as problems for research.

Standpoint epistemology holds that the knowledge available to a particular role must be developed in the light of a political commitment. For gender, race, and class standpoints, the commitment to social justice illuminates the knowledge available from the perspective of the social role. The political commitment is essential because when a social role is oppressed, the occupants tend to adopt the oppressor's view of themselves. Indeed, doing so can be a good survival strategy. A political commitment to justice helps those in the oppressed role see that they make an important contribution, and that their understanding of the social world might have some validity. Nurses, too, are committed to social justice, but justice and equality are not the political values that leverage the epistemic privilege of the nursing standpoint.

Nurse scholars must seek to promote the value of nursing practice (Meleis, 1992, p. 113). They must be committed to the idea that nursing makes a difference to health care. As Coombs' study showed, nursing work is often invisible (Coombs, 2004, Chapter 6). The nurse creates an environment where the physicians' treatment can work. This requires knowledge of health, but nursing expertise is taken for granted. In Coombs' study, both physicians and nurses treated nursing knowledge as a second-class form of knowledge. They did not appreciate the significance of the nurses' contribution to the total care of the patient. The fundamental value of nursing research, then, must be to make this knowledge explicit, to develop it, and to show its essential contribution to our understanding of human health. This value has always been a part of nursing research, even if its importance has not been appreciated. Throughout the twentieth century, nursing research has aimed to get nursing the kind of recognition it deserves. Indeed, nursing knowledge has been so undervalued that it has often been a struggle to get nurses and other health professionals to recognize that there is something for nurse researchers to investigate. Once we undertake the commitment to valorize nursing practice, the epistemic privilege of the nursing standpoint can emerge.

The philosophical questions revisited

Chapter 3 articulated four philosophical questions that underlay the theory–practice gap:

1. How is the knowledge developed in the discipline of nursing related to the professional practice of nursing?

2. What is nursing's unique area of intellectual expertise?
3. How do the values that inform nursing practice relate to nursing research and theory?
4. What is the character of scientific theories?

The idea of a nursing standpoint answers question (3) directly, and in doing so it suggests answers to questions (1) and (2). Understood as based on an epistemic standpoint, the discipline of nursing arguably has the potential to develop unique knowledge of human health. It has this potential because nurses have a role within health care that gives them a privileged perspective on a range of issues. The discipline of nursing develops and refines this epistemic perspective through commitment to both the values implicit in nursing practice and to the valorization of that practice. The values of practice inform research by directing the specific problems and questions of nursing research (cf. Question 3). Nursing's unique area of expertise is therefore exactly the knowledge necessary for practice (cf. Question 2). The discipline is given its unity through its commitment to the profession. Since nursing research and theory development begin with the problems of professional practice, nursing knowledge is closely tied to needs of practice (cf. Question 1). Arguably, this is a much closer relationship than that envisioned in the consensus model of the discipline. On that view, the discipline of nursing investigates an abstract and general domain, and applications to practice are derived from general theories. The nursing standpoint turns this model upside down. Disciplinary knowledge is always in the service of the profession.

Questions and concerns

Treating nursing knowledge as a standpoint epistemology opens a new perspective on some fundamental philosophical questions about nursing. The following chapters will be devoted to exploring the prospects and possibilities of the nursing standpoint. Before moving on, however, it will be useful to address a couple of objections that arise at the outset.

What is the nursing role?

Talk of *the* nursing standpoint might be taken to suggest that there is only one nursing role and only one place that nurses fit into the health care hierarchy. But, of course, professional nurses do all sorts of different jobs. They work in administration, public health, education, home care, clinics, hospital wards, and so on. And within these areas, nurses with different levels of training have different kinds of responsibility. Indeed, it has been a very difficult challenge for nurse scholars to find a definition of nursing or to stake out the boundaries of the profession. One might argue that there is no specific role for nurses in health care. Hence, there is no nursing standpoint.

In the early years, feminist standpoint theorists faced very similar questions. In Chapter 5, we saw how some early theorists tended to write as if there were essential characteristics to being female. The critique of this idea showed that standpoint epistemology does not presuppose an essential, timeless character to being female (or black, or a member of the working class). There may be many ways of performing gender, and the boundaries of the role may be under constant negotiation (Butler, 1990). This entails that the potential for an epistemically privileged standpoint on gender and society does not come automatically to any woman. The question is whether the role occupied by a particular woman meets the conditions for an epistemic standpoint. Just as there is no single role for women in our society, there are many ways to be a nurse. A nursing standpoint need not (and should not) presuppose that there is a single role for nurses. It is sufficient for a nursing standpoint epistemology that there be people who are employed to be, treated as, and undertake the responsibilities of, nurses. The processes of education and licensure give "the" nursing role all the stability and coherence it needs. Indeed, because the boundaries of professional nursing are policed by registration and licensure, the nursing role has substantially more stability and coherence than race, class, or gender as grounds for standpoint epistemology.

How are the boundaries of the profession determined?

A second important concern arises from the way a nursing standpoint epistemology makes the discipline depend on the profession. Economic, legal, and social pressures influence the character and boundaries of professional practice. As we saw in Chapter 1, nurse scholars in the late 1950s and early 1960s were concerned that nurses were losing their core mission. Nurses were being pushed up into managerial roles, and others were taking over direct patient care. Nurses sought to develop an academic discipline because they thought that a distinct area of intellectual expertise would help them resist inappropriate changes to nursing roles and to advance appropriate ones (Johnson, 1959a; Schlotfeld, 1960). The discipline should govern nursing, they thought, because only by doing so can the profession be defended. The nursing standpoint inverts the relationship between the profession and the discipline, and by doing so, it seems to rob the discipline of the power to determine the proper role of professional nurses in health care.

In response, a proponent of the nursing standpoint can agree that it is very important for the discipline to provide resources in the arguments about how (or how not) to change the nursing role. In the early years of nursing research, the profession was just beginning to assert its autonomy. Nurse leaders faced a chicken-and-egg kind of problem. Should the boundaries of practice be determined, and then topics for research be chosen? Or should the proper topics of research be fixed, and then the boundaries of practice set? Now, 50 years later, the profession (in the United States, at least) is more comfortable in its autonomy, and nursing has a well-established research enterprise. Nursing is now sufficiently established that it can afford the luxury of a nuanced view. According to the nursing standpoint, the profession and the discipline have a dynamic relationship. The charge of the discipline is to respond to problems of practice. Good nursing research ultimately contributes to better practice, and it thereby constitutes the knowledge base for the profession. The discipline shapes practice by developing the intellectual expertise claimed by professional nurses; the profession shapes the discipline by setting the problems with which it is to be concerned. As nurses well know, the profession of nursing exists in a social, legal, and economic context. Nurses are under pressure to change their professional responsibilities in one way or another. The expertise provided by the discipline is one (important) part of the response to these pressures. Indeed, a disciplinary knowledge base that is tightly linked to practice is in a better position to respond to social or economic pressures than a discipline where theory is regarded as irrelevant to practice.

Qualitative or quantitative?

The difference between qualitative and quantitative research has not figured in the discussion so far. For many nurse scholars, this distinction is a crucial feature of the discipline. Since qualitative perspectives have not been explicitly mentioned, the suspicion that only quantitative research and theory is being considered may arise. The differences between qualitative and quantitative research will be discussed in Part IV. For now, it must suffice to remark that a nursing standpoint should have neither a qualitative nor a quantitative bias. Qualitative research provides information about patients' experiences and their perspective on health, health care, nursing, and so on. This information is useful to both to professional nurses and nurse researchers engaged in related projects. Qualitative research is therefore a legitimate and important form of research, according to nursing standpoint theory.

Is nursing an applied science?

A related concern is that by requiring nursing research and theory to be responsive to the problems of practice, all research would have to be intervention and outcome oriented. Is there any room for theory at all, not to mention nursing history or philosophy, within the nursing discipline? To say that nursing research and theory development must *begin* from nurses' lives does not restrict nurse scholarship to the immediate problems of nursing. Effectively addressing most nursing problems will take substantial theorizing about the relevant biology, pharmacology, psychology, sociology, education theory, and so on. While it might be possible in the short run to address nursing problems piecemeal, better long-run results will come from systematic and broadly tested theories. While nursing philosophy and history do not address the immediate demands of practice, they are important sources of ideas and information that shape theories. These points are difficult to see as long as we remain committed to the conception of theory that has dominated nursing since the 1970s. Chapter 10 will critique this view of theories, and subsequent chapters will develop an alternative.

Finally, some may worry that, without a unifying metaparadigm, nursing will turn into an applied science. Nurses have resisted this because it seems to trivialize the discipline. Moreover, the nursing standpoint seems to be promiscuous about the use of theory from other disciplines. Many will object that such a view will be conceptually and empirically incoherent (e.g., Cody, 1999). Like the previous concern, this depends on the dominant ideas about the structure of nursing theory, ideas that have their origins in the consensus of the 1970s. As we saw in Chapter 2, this consensus held that disciplines were unified by their highest level laws, and the concepts that appeared in those laws determined the possible content of middle-range theories. The application of theory to practice, then, is analogous to engineering. When an engineer sets out to design a bridge, the task requires knowledge of the general principles of physics, material science, and so on. The engineer plugs values into the equations, and works out the dimensions of the bridge supports. Analogously, grand theory in nursing was to entail middle-range theories, which could be applied to practice. The concern about nursing being an applied science depends on this engineering analogy, and it is only as compelling as the philosophical model of theory on which it is based. Again, subsequent chapters will argue against this dominant model, both in its conception of theory structure and its understanding of scientific concepts. With the philosophical blinders removed, we will be able to see the shape of nursing science more clearly.

Conclusion: science and standpoint

The unique character of nursing knowledge—the intellectual foundation of the discipline—is found in the perspective on human health available to professional nurses. The nursing standpoint thus points toward answers to three of the four philosophical questions from Chapter 3. The questions and concerns we have been discussing highlight the deep importance of the fourth question: What is the character of scientific theories? The standpoint picture is a bottom-up account of nursing knowledge. The alternative, top-down account is strongly supported by a cluster of philosophical ideas about science. To appreciate the idea of a nursing standpoint, then, we will have to carefully unpack, and then reassemble, the philosophical views about theory that have influenced nursing scholarship.

Part III
Nursing Theory and the Philosophy of Science

Introduction to Part III

In a 1973 lecture to the *American Nurses Association Nursing Research Conference*, Walker argued that the practice theorists had an overly broad conception of theory. She quoted Ellis' definition of a theory as "a coherent hypothesis, or set of hypotheses, or a concept, forming a general framework for undertaking something" (Ellis, 1969, p. 1434). She also mentioned Dickoff and James' slogan that a theory is a conceptual structure built for a purpose. Walker pointed out that these conceptions of theory are unsuitably broad. According to them, any kind of activity-directing metaphor counts as theory. For example, tennis players and golfers are sometimes told to swing through the ball, as if the ball was not there. This is a conceptual structure with the purpose of helping the player perform well. It would be absurd, however, to think of this metaphor as a scientific theory. Walker concluded that nursing should adopt a "tighter use of 'theory' more in line with its conventional use in the sciences" (Walker, [1973] 1997, p. 74). Walker's critique thus raised for nursing a fundamental question of the philosophy of science: What is a scientific theory?

Walker was among many nurse scholars in the 1970s who wanted to develop the empirical, scientific side of nursing knowledge. In their vision of the discipline, nursing was analogous to other basic sciences in the academy. Nursing would have its own conceptual apparatus, laws, and subject matter. It would develop a distinctive body of knowledge from which practitioners could draw, thus supporting nursing's claims to professionalism. In their philosophical thinking about what a basic science should be like, nurse scholars articulated views about the character of scientific theories, concepts, methods, and evidence. This philosophical view of science became the center of the 1970s consensus about the character of the nursing science.

Chapter 2 argued that nurse scholars came to regard nursing as a basic science because of a philosophy of science known as "the received view of theory." It is ironic that as nurses were discovering and adopting this view, philosophers of science were abandoning it. If, as Chapter 2 argued, the relevance gap is a consequence of the philosophy of science adopted by nurse scholars, it is crucial to understand the received view of theory, how it influenced nursing, and why philosophers rejected it. The chapters of this Part will address that task. Chapter 8 will unpack the philosophical ideas that surround the received view of theory. By necessity, this chapter will be rather detailed and technical. Chapter 9 will trace the influence of the received view on nursing scholarship. Nurse scholars have debated how this philosophy of science influenced nursing theory (Gortner, 1993; Suppe & Jacox, 1985). With the elements of the received view in hand, we will be able to show that the influence of the received view is much deeper and more pervasive than has been previously imagined. It is all the more important, then, to understand why philosophers of science rejected the received view of theory. Chapter 10 will present some of the important arguments. Since most contemporary philosophical views about science take their starting point from these criticisms, it will be important to treat the arguments in some detail. The chapters of Part IV will begin to trace the positive consequences for nursing conceptions of theory.

Logical positivism and mid-century philosophy of science

Logical positivism is not warmly remembered by contemporary scholars. Indeed, "positivist" is widely used as a term of abuse. Nonetheless, there are important historical and philosophical issues to be sorted out. The aim of this chapter will be to clearly articulate the commitments of a view of scientific theory that was prevalent in the mid-twentieth century. Once the features of this philosophy of science have been identified, we will be able to trace the relationship between the ideas of the philosophers and the ideas of nursing scholars.

Some history and terminology

One source of ambiguity about the influence of mid-century philosophy of science on nursing has been the terminological profligacy of both philosophers and nurse scholars. Terms such as "positivism," "logical positivism," "empiricism," "logical empiricism," "the received view," "postpositivism," and "realism," are used in a variety of overlapping ways.[1] To clarify these matters, we must begin with some understanding of how philosophers have used these terms to describe themselves.

Empiricism

"Empiricism," as the term will be used here, is a philosophical approach to understanding knowledge. It is one kind of position within the field of epistemology. The central commitment of empiricists is that all knowledge arises from experience. In the seventeenth and eighteenth centuries, empiricism contrasted with rationalism.

---

[1] Good discussions of empiricism and logical positivism in nursing may be found in Suppe and Jacox (1985), Jacox and Webster (1986), Gortner (1993), and Weiss (1995).

Rationalists denied that all knowledge arose from experience. They held that some knowledge could be obtained through reasoning and reflection alone, without input from observation or experiment. Empiricism, then, is the epistemological view that takes sensory experience to be the ultimate court of appeal for all claims to know about physical objects, people, and societies.[2] Moreover, empiricism is a view about our knowledge of things, not a view about what kinds of things exist. (That is to say, empiricism is an epistemology, not an ontology.) Hence, empiricism does not entail realism, materialism, or reductionism, as is sometimes suggested in nursing discussions. Some empiricists have held that our perceptions represent an external world (realism) and others have denied this (antirealism or idealism). Some empiricists have held that all real things are composites of physical atoms (materialism and reductionism). Others have held that souls are distinct from bodies (antimaterialism) and that some objects are different from the sum of their parts (antireductionism). As philosophers use the term, then, calling a view as "empiricist" merely characterizes a commitment to observation as the sole source of knowledge.

Most philosophers in the twentieth century have held that knowledge arises from experience, and in this sense, most have been empiricists. Logical positivism is a particular way of working out the commitments of empiricism. But so is phenomenology, especially in its Husserlian form. Both logical positivists and phenomenologists emphasize the importance of experience in the formation of knowledge. Their dispute is (partly) about the character of experience. The positivists wanted to think of experience as the observation of discrete qualities, such as "red," "hot," or "smooth," while the phenomenologists wanted to understand experience more organically. Logical positivists also had a view about the structure of knowledge that was different from the phenomenologists. Knowledge, they thought, was a matter of forming successively more powerful generalizations out of the raw material of observation. We will unpack this idea in some detail below.

Logical positivism

Logical positivism had its origins in a group of philosophers known as the Vienna Circle. It has also been called "logical empiricism" and simply "positivism." The height of their influence was during the 1930s and 1940s. A key commitment of the logical positivist's version of empiricism was that every meaningful statement must be verifiable. If there is no conceivable way to test whether a statement is true, the logical positivists thought, it is empty, meaningless. Since science is the form of knowledge that embodies this ideal most clearly, the logical positivists turned their attention to scientific knowledge. A distinctive feature of science is that it describes objects (such as electrons, genes, or viruses) that are not directly observable. If statements about genes were to be meaningful, they must be somehow related to statements that described possible observations. The logical positivists thus developed a philosophical understanding of science that showed how abstract theories

---

[2] Both rationalists and empiricists had ways of understanding scientific knowledge, so it would not be correct to think of empiricism as more closely aligned with the sciences than rationalism.

could be related to more concrete and testable theories, and how theories might be confirmed. Their goal was to show how statements about unobservable objects such as genes or electrons could be verified, and thus made meaningful.

As a philosophical school, logical positivism fell from favor among philosophers in the late 1950s. While philosophers rejected the main commitments of logical positivism, many aspects of the positivists' philosophy of science survived, and it survived both within philosophy and outside of it, especially in the social sciences. For this reason, philosophers of science in the 1970s began using the phrase "the received view of theory" to refer to a collection of philosophical ideas about science. In the 1950s and 1960s, not everyone who agreed with the philosophical perspective on science was also committed to the tenets of logical positivism. Karl Popper is a case in point: he explicitly rejected some of the central commitments of the logical positivists, but his view of science substantially overlapped with them.

Conceptions of theory in nursing

In the 1970s, prominent nursing scholars were remarkably consistent in their characterization of scientific theory. Consider the following quotations from works that have often been cited as authoritative:

"Nagel's[3] analysis of the cognitive status of theories indicates that all three components can usually be identified in a theory, namely, 'an abstract set of postulates which implicitly define the basic terms of the theory, a model or interpretation for the postulates, and rules of correspondence for terms in the postulates or in the theorems derived from them.'" (King, 1971, p. 13)

"Part of the definition of a theory is that it is a systematically related set of statements of propositions. This means that the propositions are deductively arranged—some basic propositions are assumed to be true. This assumption is based on what the theorist considers to be adequate empirical evidence to support the assertions made by the propositions. These basic propositions are called 'axioms.' From them, other propositions called 'theorems' are deduced." (Jacox, 1974, p. 412)

"From a philosophic point of view, a theory is a set of sentences whose purpose is to explain. The specific vocabulary of these sentences includes primitive terms. Hempel (p. 183),[4] in his discussion of scientific concepts and theories, points out that 'many of the sentences of a theory are derivable from others by means of the principles of deductive logic (and the definitions of the defined terms); but on pain of a vicious circle or an infinite regress in the deduction, not all of the theoretical sentences can be thus established. Hence, the set of sentences asserted by theory falls into two subsets: primitive sentences, or postulates (also called axioms), and derivative sentences, or theorems.'" (Riehl & Roy, 1974, p. 3)

---

[3] King is quoting Nagel (1961, p. 106).
[4] Riehl and Roy are quoting Hempel (1965, p. 183).

"The central core of a theory consists of its postulates. These are statements of general truth that serve as essential premises for whatever is being investigated. Postulates are usually stated as generalizations which are consistent with scientific evidence related to one's research problem. They form the essential presuppositions from which hypotheses are deduced and tested. Rogers (1970, pp. 46–47), for example, in developing her theoretical basis of nursing, identified four essential postulates about man." (Silva, 1977, p. 61)

"Concepts are connected in a theory by verbal or mathematical statements called propositions. Propositions describe the theoretical linkages between concepts. Two types of propositions are generally found in a theory. Axioms, or initial propositions, are the starting points for derivations; they are not to be tested, but rather taken as givens in the theory. In contrast, postulates, also called deduced propositions or theorems, are statements of supposition regarding the type of relation between the concepts of the theory. A theory's explanatory power is found in its postulates." (Fawcett, 1978, p. 51)

A number of themes run through these quotations. First, they take the core of a theory to be a set of postulates (or axioms). Second, the postulates contain basic (or primitive) terms that are implicitly defined by the postulates. Third, from the postulates a number of theorems are derived. In these passages, the authors pick up one of the distinctive ideas of the logical positivist philosophy of science: they are treating scientific theories as analogous to mathematical axiom systems.

The logical rigor of mathematics has fascinated intellectuals since ancient times, and Euclid's *Elements* has often served as a model of theory. Euclid arranged geometric knowledge systematically by specifying the definitions, postulates, and axioms at the outset. All of the truths of geometry were then proven using only these resources. Newton adopted the same model of theory when he presented his three laws of motion and derived from them the explanation of many well-known phenomena. Until the nineteenth century, Euclidean geometry was the only fully axiomatized mathematical theory. In the late nineteenth century, axioms of arithmetic were developed and alternative axioms for geometry were discovered. Logic was given an axiomatic formulation too. These developments in mathematics and logic permitted philosophers and scientists to imagine that all theory should be understood axiomatically, and it gave them rigorous ways of representing the logical structure of scientific theory. One of the most significant contributions of the logical positivists was to work out how modern logic might be used to represent scientific theories as axiomatic systems. The quotations above show how nursing too was caught up with this image of theory.

Theories and axiom systems

Euclid and Newton

To understand what it means to treat a scientific theory as an axiomatic formal system, it might be helpful to turn to the source: Eucild's *Elements*. Euclid systematized the geometric knowledge of his day by forming a set of first principles, or axioms.[5] They were "first" in the sense that they were used as premises in Euclid's proofs, but not themselves ever proven. Examples of Euclid's axioms are that *all right angles are equal to each other*, and that *for any point and radius, a circle can be described*. Using the axioms, Euclid could prove all the truths of geometry: for example, that the interior angles of any triangle are equal to two right angles (180°) or that, any three points (not falling on a line) can be connected as part of a circle. These latter propositions are *theorems* of geometry. Theorems are proven from the axioms using deductive logic. The distinctive feature of deductive logic is that, in a good deductive argument (technically, a "valid argument"), it is impossible for the premises to be true and the conclusion false. This means that if Euclid's axioms are true, then the theorems must be true too. Figuratively speaking, the truth of the theorems flows from the truth of the axioms. And so knowledge of the axioms is, in a sense, knowledge of the whole domain. The beauty of an axiomatic system is that it condenses a vast body of truths into a surveyable number of elementary truths. Euclid used 10 axioms (and a substantial number of definitions) to prove well over 400 theorems. Moreover, because some theorems were used as premises in subsequent proofs, the logical dependencies among the various geometric truths could be illuminated.

Euclid's axiomatic treatment of geometry has often been emulated in the sciences, but Isaac Newton's *Principia Mathematica* is perhaps the most famous. Newton postulated three laws of motion, and with the aid of the newly developed mathematics of the calculus, he showed how a large number of often observed facts about moving bodies could be deduced from his laws. For example, a stone whirled on a string moves in a circle. When released, the stone will fly away at a tangent to the circle. Newton could deduce this behavior from his laws by treating the string as exerting a force on the stone. When the string is released, the law of inertia (objects in motion tend to stay in motion) entails that it will move in a straight line from the point of release. Descriptions of observable regularities (like a stone flung by a sling) were thus treated as theorems.

Challenges to an axiomatic treatment of theory

Treating a scientific theory as an axiomatic system like Euclid's *Elements* raises several philosophical questions. Most prominent among them: Why should we think that the axioms are true? In Euclid's case, the axioms seem obvious or self-evident: for example, the whole is greater than the part (Common notion 5) or that all right angles equal one another (Postulate 4). In Newton's theory, the laws of motion are far from obvious. Moreover, it is possible to think of the theorems of Euclid's geometry as true simply in virtue of the definitions and axioms (and the logical positivists did so). As subsequent mathematicians discovered, the axioms can be changed, and different "nonEuclidean" geometrical systems emerge. Newton's theory, however,

---

[5] Euclid distinguished between definitions, postulates, and common notions. We will follow contemporary practice and treat all first principles as "axioms." All translations are taken from the Heath edition (Heath, 1952).

is supposed to be a description of the physical world. Newton's laws are not true by convention. If they are true, it is because they correctly represent hidden forces and relationships. Moreover, Euclid's definitions seem uncontroversial, for example, that a triangle has three sides. By contrast, Newton's theory used new concepts, such as inertia, acceleration, mass, and gravity, and these terms were supposed to pick out hidden objects and properties. How are these new terms of the theory to be defined? And why accept one definition rather than another?

The logical positivists approached these questions from an empiricist point of view. All knowledge arises from experience, according to empiricism, so the problem was to show how an axiomatic system could be justified on the basis of experience. Their idea was that a theory is justified by its observational consequences. The reason why we accept Newton's laws is that a wide variety of explanations can be derived from them. The axioms of a scientific theory must therefore entail observable consequences. For a scientific theory, then, there is an important difference between the axioms (or postulates) and the theorems. The axioms cannot be tested directly. The theorems of a scientific theory should refer to observable objects and properties so that their truth or falsity can be determined by observation.

The positivists' ideas about theory testing faced a substantial hurdle: the central propositions of a scientific theory usually refer to objects or properties that are not observable. Viruses are too small, the solar system is too big, and the signing of the *Magna Carta* is too historically remote to observe. Newton used the idea of force in his second law, and he was criticized for introducing "occult" entities into science. Somehow, axioms about unobservables need to logically entail theorems about observables. But how can the theoretical terms in the axioms be connected to the observational terms of the theorems?

Implicit definition

A similar problem about definition had long been recognized in Euclid's *Elements*. Euclid defined a line as a "breadthless length," yet he did not go on to define "breadth" and "length." Euclid's definitions depended on antecedent knowledge; the reader must already know what these terms mean. But the point of an axiomatic treatment is that knowledge of the first principles is sufficient for the knowledge of the whole body of truths. Anything necessary for the proof of the theorems must be incorporated into the first principles. Doing so, however, makes the definitions circular. Like the words in the dictionary, if every word is given an explicit definition, each is ultimately defined by reference to the others. The only way to avoid circularity is to leave some terms without explicit definitions. In the jargon of the time, these words were called "primitive terms." The problem faced by the logical positivists about the theoretical terms in scientific axioms was thus captured in the question: How can primitive terms be justified?

In the late nineteenth century, mathematicians found a way out of this conundrum. They identified the meaning of primitive terms with the consequences of the axioms of which they were part. The root idea is that meaning of the word "line" should capture all of the essential properties of lines. Such properties are expressed in the theorems. Since the theorems are logical consequences of the axioms, the axioms already express all of the properties of the primitive terms. So, for example, imagine removing the axioms that use the word "circle" from Euclid's axioms. Using the reduced set, there are still a number of theorems that can be proven (e.g., theorems about triangles). Not as many, of course: the set of theorems that can be proven with the word "circle" (call this set T) is bigger than the set of theorems that can be proven without it (call it T^*). The meaning of the word "circle" in Euclid's system is the difference between T and T^*. This difference captures all of the essential properties of circles without requiring an explicit definition. The primitive terms in the axioms, therefore, do not need explicit definitions. They are implicitly defined by their role in the axioms.

In their discussions of theory structure, King uses the phrase "implicitly define" (King, 1971, p. 13) and Riehl and Roy talk about "primitive terms" (Riehl & Roy, 1974, p. 3). They are using these phrases in the way that the logical positivists did. The logical positivists solved the problem of how to define theoretical terms (which referred to unobservable entities) by applying the mathematical idea of an implicit definition. The ideas of force or mass, as they appear in Newton's theory, is just the difference that such terms make to the theory. An important difference between Newton's and Euclid's theories, of course, is that Newton's theory has observable consequences. While force and mass are not directly observable (remember that mass is not the same as weight), the axioms of which they are a part have observable consequences. Indeed, since each term makes a specific contribution to the explanatory power of the theory, the meaning of a theoretical term can be identified with its observable consequences.

Theory structure: the received view

The received view of theory is a response to the problem of how to understand theories as axiomatic systems within an empiricist epistemological framework. If all knowledge arises from experience, then the basis for scientific knowledge must be observation. Observation therefore must play a special role in science. It must be the ultimate court of appeal for theory choice. If the choice of theories is to be objective, observations must not be biased toward one theory or another. The positivists responded to the need for unbiased observations by strictly distinguishing between terms that referred to observable objects and properties and those terms that referred to unobservable, or "theoretical," entities. They sometimes treated these as different vocabularies or languages. Examples of the observational vocabulary would be words such as "brown," "cat," "weighs two kilograms," or "is moving at one meter per minute." Examples of the theoretical vocabulary would be words such as "black hole," "virus," or "oxygen." If a sentence is formulated in the observational vocabulary, then, under the right conditions, its truth or falsity can be directly determined. Thus, the truth of "the cat is brown" or "the cat weighs two kilograms" can be determined by observing the specified cat. Sentences that deploy theoretical vocabulary cannot be verified directly. Whether a compound contains oxygen, or whether a person is infected with a particular virus, cannot be directly observed. The problem of science, from the empiricist point of view, is to show how statements in the theoretical language could be supported (justified) by statements of the observational language.

According to the received view, a scientific theory has the following structure:

1. A theoretical vocabulary.
2. A set of axioms, expressed in the theoretical vocabulary.
3. A set of bridge laws that relate theoretical terms to observation terms.

In a scientific theory, each of the axioms represents a law of nature. The primitive theoretical terms are implicitly defined by their role in the axioms, and other theoretical terms can be defined by combining the primitive terms. The "bridge laws" (also sometimes called "correspondence rules") are necessary because a theory composed in a theoretical vocabulary alone would not be testable. The theoretical terms are not observable, and axioms expressed entirely in theoretical terms would have no observational consequences. Therefore, there must be a set of statements that link the observational and the theoretical vocabularies. This is the function of the bridge laws. With the addition of bridge laws, the theorems include observational statements that can be directly tested. According to the received view of theory, *all* properly scientific theories have this structure. And since scientific knowledge is knowledge of theory, all scientific knowledge has this structure as well.

Theoretical and experimental laws

The received view of theory has important consequences for the way in which theories are related. Philosophers in this tradition typically distinguished between "theoretical" and "experimental" laws (Nagel, 1961, p. 80). The first principles of a scientific theory would have to be very abstract and general laws. Much scientific research, however, aims at discovering observable regularities. Boyle's law, for example, was discovered in the seventeenth century. It holds that, when a given volume of gas is held at constant temperature, its pressure and volume are inversely proportional; as the pressure increases, the volume decreases, and vice versa. It was 200 years before there was a generally accepted theoretical understanding of why gases behaved in this way. Boyle's law thus seems to have a different character than the laws that serve as the first principles of a theory. It is a simple empirical generalization (or experimental law). Scientific research, according to the received view, thus works in two directions. Empirical research aims to inductively discover regularities in the observable world. Such generalizations would be couched in the observation language. Theoretical research is more speculative. It postulates general laws and formulates them with the aid of a theoretical vocabulary. The goal of science, on this view, is to connect the two sorts of laws by deducing the empirical laws from the theory.

To see how science was supposed to relate theoretical and empirical laws, consider again the example of Newton's theory. A famous application of Newton's theory was to explain the ocean tides. The tides, of course, were a well-known phenomenon. People who live near the sea have long known how to predict the strength and rhythm of the tides. Prior to Newton, then, there were well-known empirical generalizations (or experimental laws) about the tides. Newton's three laws of motion speak only about forces and motions; they say nothing about bodies of water. Newton and later scientists were able to show how the tides were the result of the sun and the moon's gravitational pull on the ocean's water. Gravity pulls the water toward the moon, and as the earth rotates, the wave moves across the surface of the earth. In the eighteenth century, scientists working with Newton's laws of motion were able to describe these effects with mathematical precision, ultimately deducing the well-known empirical generalizations about the tides from Newton's fundamental laws. To make their derivations, however, they had to add premises about the mass of the moon, the sun, and the ocean water (among many other contingent, empirical facts). Notice how this theory of the tides relies on both the fundamental laws of Newton's theory and specific, local information. Tides only happen when a planet has sufficiently large and deep bodies of liquid upon its surface, and only when the planet has a sufficiently large moon. Adding such local information to the fundamental laws of Newton's theory creates another theory—a middle-range theory—that has more local application, more precise predictions about specific events, and is more testable.

The hierarchy of theory

It is natural, on the received view, to think of different theories as related in a hierarchy. At the highest level are the fundamental laws. They provide the implicit definitions of the fundamental concepts, and they are the ultimate premises for all derivations. Lower level theories are derived by adding more specific information to the general theory. (In the example of the tides, this was information about the volume of earth's oceans, distance to the sun, and so on.) From these lower level (middle-range) theories, the experimental laws or empirical generalizations can be derived. Within a given discipline, then, theories can be imagined as falling within a hierarchy.

Whether the disciplines themselves formed a hierarchy was an important question for mid-century philosophers of science. Some argued that the sciences could be unified into a single system (Oppenheim & Putnam, 1958). The most general laws (presumably laws of physics) would be the first principles of all knowledge. The other laws of chemistry, biology, psychology, sociology, and so on, would be derived from the fundamental laws in the manner of middle-range theories. In this way, all of the sciences would be reduced to physics. Other philosophers were more cautious (e.g., Nagel, 1961). As philosophers of science explored the details of the relationship among, say, laws of chemistry and laws of biology, they found that the conditions for a full reduction of one domain to another were difficult, if not impossible, to meet. Through the 1950s and 1960s, the problem of reductionism was debated within the framework of empiricism and the received view of theory.

Explanation and confirmation

Explanation

When an empirical regularity (like the rhythm of the tides) or an experimental law (like Boyle's gas law) is shown to be a consequence of more fundamental laws, it seems appropriate to say that the phenomenon has been *explained*. When eighteenth century physicists deduced tidal patterns from Newton's laws, they explained why the ocean has tides. Or again, the law of gravity explains why an apple falls toward the earth. Mid-century philosophers of science embraced this idea, and they used it to provide an account of explanation that was a natural extension of their view of theory structure. Carl Hempel did the most to develop this idea of explanation (Hempel, 1965). According to Hempel, an explanation has the following elements:

1. An event or empirical regularity to be explained.
2. A number of general laws.
3. A set of initial conditions.

Following Hempel's terminology, philosophers of science call the event or regularity to be explained the "explanandum." The laws and initial conditions do the explaining, so (2) and (3) together are called the "explanans." An explanation needs both (2) and (3) because the laws are general. The initial conditions describe the causes or initial state of the system. Where the laws are expressed as mathematical formulas, the initial conditions provide values for some of the variables.

According to Hempel, an event or empirical regularity is explained when it is shown to be the logical consequence of a set of laws and initial conditions. Suppose, for example, we want to explain why the falling apple had a particular velocity when it hits the ground. Newton's second law states that $F = ma$; force equals mass times acceleration, and acceleration is defined as change in velocity over time ($a = dv/dt$). Given the law and the definition, velocity at the time the apple hits the ground can be calculated if we know the initial conditions. In this case, those are the mass of the apple, m, and the gravitational force, F, acting upon the apple, and the amount of time it falls. The calculation of the velocity explains why the apple hit the ground with a particular velocity. Because an explanation was the *deduction* of the explanandum from *laws*, Hempel called his view the "deductive-nomological" conception of explanation.[6]

Hempel's work on explanation neatly dovetailed with the view of theories as axiomatic systems of laws. Explanation is, arguably, one of the goals of scientific inquiry. On Hempel's view, a theory was by its very nature explanatory. The deduction of experimental laws from fundamental laws (or the deduction of one theory from another) was an explanation of them. It showed how observable regularities were the consequence of deeper facts about the world. Conversely, explanations

---

[6] Hempel also developed a view about explanations that employ statistical or probabilistic relationships. This form of explanation will not figure in our discussion, so it is omitted here.

required laws, and all laws were components of theory. So, the scientific enterprise of explaining natural and social phenomena required the development of theories.

Theory testing

One crucial feature of scientific inquiry has not yet been discussed. How are scientific theories tested? On what grounds do we judge a theory to be justified, and when do we reject or modify the theory? As we have already seen, empiricism requires that theories be tested by observation. On the received view of theories, this idea has a very simple application. To test a theory, a proposition must be derived that can be observed to be true or false. This would be a hypothesis or prediction. The deduction of a hypothesis will require correspondence rules (or bridge laws) to relate the observational vocabulary to the theoretical vocabulary of the fundamental laws. Moreover, it will require substantial claims about the local conditions—in other words, it will typically require middle-range theory too. In its essential structure, then, theory testing has the same form as explanation: it is the deduction of an observable proposition from laws and initial conditions. The difference is that in explanation, the explanandum is already known. (We know the apple falls, but why?) In prediction, the hypothesis is not yet known to be true or false.

Within the framework of the received view of theories, there was a dispute about the character of theory testing. Some held that all theory testing was deductive. Sir Karl Popper was the most important proponent of this view (Popper, 1963, 1968). Popper held that theory testing proceeded entirely through the logic of falsification. This meant that to test a theory, a hypothesis would be derived from the laws. If the hypothesis was observed to be false, then the theory must be mistaken in some way. As a matter of logic, if a false statement is validly derived from a set of premises, then one of those premises must be false.[7] A scientist can thus be certain that a theory is false (i.e., it has at least one false law) if the hypothesis fails. Unfortunately, there is no corresponding certainty that a theory is true. A false proposition can have logical consequences that are true. For example, I might postulate the "law" that persons who eat cheese never get lung cancer. On the basis of this "law," I could predict that my cheese-eating friend, Kurt, will never get lung cancer. Kurt may never be afflicted with the dreaded disease, but that does little to show that my "theory" is true. Perhaps Kurt and I were just lucky. Popper thus concluded that theories are never positively verified or confirmed. The task of a scientist, according to Popper, is to submit her theories to severe tests; to try to falsify them. She will never prove her theories to be true. The best she can say is that her theories have not yet been proven false.[8]

---

[7] By definition, an argument is valid if there is no situation where the premises are true and the conclusion false. If the argument is valid and has a false conclusion, then the premises cannot all be true.

[8] Popper had a view of scientific progress that fits with his falsificationist view, but the details are unnecessary for our discussion.

Against Popper, other philosophers of science tried to show that theories could get positive, inductive support (Goodman, 1955; Carnap, 1962; Hempel, 1965). These philosophers agreed that a false hypothesis showed that one of the laws of the theory must be false. They disagreed with Popper about whether a true hypothesis had value. They tried various ways to conceptualize (and quantify) the degree to which a successful prediction supported the theory from which it was derived. The details of these views are not crucial for our present purposes. The take-home lesson of this dispute is that theory testing, on the received view, was a matter of deducing hypotheses from the fundamental laws of the theory. In this way, a theory is tested by its observational consequences.

Conclusion: logical positivism and scientific knowledge

The received view of theory was thus at the core of a systematic understanding of the scientific enterprise. It treated scientific theories as axiomatic systems of laws, and it showed how reference to unobservable entities might be made respectable within an empiricist epistemology. It also provided accounts of scientific explanation and theory testing. Arguably, these are central aspects of scientific inquiry. The received view of theories therefore had important consequences for the way in which philosophers thought about scientific knowledge.

For the logical positivists, the main questions about science were epistemological: What is scientific knowledge and what makes scientific knowledge possible? They took their philosophy of science to answer both questions. Scientific knowledge is knowledge of the fundamental laws of nature. These are expressed as the first principles or axioms of a theory. Scientific knowledge becomes possible because observational statements are derived from the laws, and these observations can be tested. A good theory is one with explanatory power, and this is a matter of deducing explanations from the laws. The primary activity of science, then, is the production and testing of theory.

The received view of theory has consequences for the understanding of scientific disciplines: the differences among disciplines correspond to differences among theories. If a scientific theory is defined by its fundamental axioms, then different theories must have different axioms. Central concepts are implicitly defined by the axioms, so theories encompass a body of unique concepts. The academic disciplines, as they evolved in the twentieth century, have coalesced around fundamental theories—theories of mechanics, and dynamics in physics; theories of compounds in chemistry; theories of living things in biology. Scientific disciplines, according to the logical positivists' conception of science, were thus aligned with theories. A discipline that constituted a basic science should have its own body of laws. Since fundamental concepts are implicitly defined by the laws, a basic science would have unique concepts. A proper scientific discipline, according to the received view of scientific theory, would therefore be a basic science with its own theories and conceptual framework.

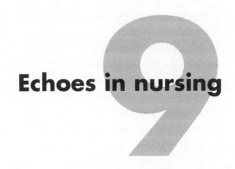

Echoes in nursing

Did logical positivism influence nursing?

It is easy to see the influence of logical positivism and the received view of theories in the quotations from King, Riehl and Roy, Jacox, Silva, and Fawcett in Chapter 8. The account of theory in King's *Toward a Theory for Nursing* (1971), for example, is based directly on Nagel (1961). King contended that a theory is composed of a set of "postulates," that the set of postulates "implicitly define" the basic concepts of the theory, and that the postulates must "have a relationship to observable phenomena," a relationship she called a "correspondence rule" (King, 1971, pp. 13–15). Similar points could be made about each of the essays quoted above, as well as many other nursing essays and textbooks on theory. It is clear that, at least in the 1970s, the received view of theory was profoundly influential in nursing.

One might think that the influence of the received view on nursing was limited to the 1970s. After all, nurse scholars were also influenced by Kuhn ([1962] 1970), Lauden (1977), Suppe (Suppe & Jacox, 1985; Suppe, 1989) and other postpositivist philosophers of science. Watson's landmark essay, "Nursing's scientific quest" (1981), included a substantial discussion of the received view and how it had fallen from favor among philosophers of science. She went on to chart a course for nursing science that led out of the positivist philosophical framework. Given the subsequent adoption of ideas from phenomenology, critical theory, and postmodernism, one might think that nursing's entanglement with the received view of theories was nothing more than a youthful flirtation. And yet, young love can shape later relationships. The received view of theories continues to exert a deep and thoroughgoing influence on discussions of nursing science.

Three kinds of influence

The discussion of how logical positivism influenced nursing has been vexed:

> *"Suppe and Jacox's (1985) essay on philosophic influences on nursing theory development appears to be the major source for contentions that nursing theory has been influenced by positivism. Whether this contention of influence is accurate, despite assertions in our literature that it is, would depend on evidence that we don't have and preferably would have to be garnered from the theorists themselves. At the conference where this paper was originally presented, both Hesook Suzie Kim and Callista Roy were present; neither acknowledged the supposed influence of positivism on their own writings."* (Gortner, 1993, p. 481)

In this passage, Gortner interpreted influence as an intentional matter. Nurse authors were influenced only insofar as they consciously and intentionally applied positivist doctrine to their work. Gortner may be correct in her assertion that these nurse scholars did not self-consciously adopt the program of logical positivism. But ideas may be important and influential even when they are not deliberately adopted. There are at least two other ways in which the influence of ideas may be identified.

Influence of ideas can be textually maintained. In this sense of "influence," authors are influenced when they draw on (by positive citation or quotation) works in the logical positivist tradition. Prominent writers in the logical positivist and "the received view of theory" tradition include Hempel (1965), Nagel (1961), Popper (1963), and Reichenbach (1951). Insofar as essays by nurse scholars cite these texts as authorities, and those nursing essays are themselves cited as authorities, the received view of theory can be said to be influential.

Another sense of "influence" is less historical and more philosophical. The logical positivists were refining views of scientific theory that were common in the nineteenth and twentieth centuries. So, even if nurse scholars did not cite the logical positivists, they may have shared important ideas with them. Nurse scholars would be influenced by the received view of theory insofar as they developed substantially similar ideas. This third sense is philosophically important because the received view of theory has been sharply criticized. If the ideas are very similar, then the criticism might extend to nursing views of theory too.

There are, then, three ways in which the received view of theory might have been influential on nursing scholarship. Nurse scholars may have intentionally adopted the ideas, they may have transmitted them through authoritative quotation and citation, or they may have simply shared ideas that were in common use. Even if nurse scholars did not deliberately adopt a positivist perspective on science, a cursory look at the nursing metatheoretical literature shows that they were influenced in the second and third senses. Not only did key essays about nursing theory cite philosophers who defended the received view of theory (Hempel, Nagel, and Popper were favorites), but also ideas associated with the received view of theory were central to the nursing consensus of the 1970s. And this is not merely a historical curiosity: these ideas about theory continue to shape the nursing literature.

Positivism and the critique of nursing metatheory

Since the word "positivism" has become a pejorative in many quarters, tracing an intellectual affinity between logical positivism and nursing theory will be taken by some to be an indictment. But it would be unfair and superficial to criticize nurse scholars on such grounds. The received view of theory represents a way of thinking about science that was common—among scientists as well as philosophers—in the nineteenth and twentieth centuries. The logical positivist contribution was to develop this view and crystallize its commitments. But as so often happens, when the ideas are made fully explicit, we can clearly see their defects. The received view of theory was abandoned by many philosophers of science because of specific arguments against it.

The important issue, then, is whether criticisms of the received view in the philosophy of science also cut against nursing ideas. Literature in nursing metatheory shows the marks of the received view of theory in three areas: (1) the perceived need for a metaparadigm, (2) the commitment to levels of theory, and (3) the concern that borrowed theories dilute the discipline. Each of these ideas reflects aspects of the received view of theory that have been criticized in the philosophy of science. The historical question of the influence of the received view is thus only a means of reaching deeper and more important questions about nursing science.

The metaparadigm of nursing

The question of how nursing is to be unified or defined runs throughout the nursing literature. We saw in Part I how it became particularly pressing as nursing developed into a discipline. In the 1950s and 1960s, the question was typically phrased as a problem of finding a nursing philosophy or a definition of nursing (Johnson, 1959a; Henderson, 1966). These scholars sought to delineate the proper scope of the nursing profession. During this period, research by nurses tended to be closely related to nursing practice. Hence, if the boundaries of nursing practice were secured by a nursing philosophy, the unity of the discipline would also be ensured.

In the early 1980s, the character of this discussion changed. Fawcett's essay "The metaparadigm of nursing: present status and future refinements" (1984) proposed the idea that the unity of nursing should be provided by a set of concepts and themes.[1] She drew the concepts of person, health, environment, and nursing from existing research (1984, p. 3). The three themes were taken from Donaldson and Crowley (1978). The function of the metaparadigm, as Fawcett saw it, was to "identify the phenomena central to the discipline of nursing in an abstract, global manner" (1984, p. 4). After the publication of Fawcett's essay, most nursing literature took it for granted that the discipline of nursing required a metaparadigm. Authors who commented on the metaparadigm did not ask whether it was the

---

[1] Important precursors to Fawcett's work included Hardy (1978), Smith (1979), and Flaskerud and Halloran (1980).

appropriate way to unify the discipline. Rather, subsequent essays about nursing's metaparadigm concerned the definition of the concepts (person, health, environment, and nursing), whether all the concepts were really necessary, and whether additional concepts might be required.

Validity of the metaparadigm

Fawcett's seminal essay is remarkable in two respects. In a response to Fawcett's essay, June Brody pointed out that Fawcett made no attempt to establish that the metaparadigm had "external validity" (1984, p. 88). The bulk of the essay is devoted to showing how various nursing studies from the 1970s and 1980s could be fit into the concepts and themes. But, Brody remarked, "surely a metaparadigm is more than a systematic identification and formulation of concepts and themes" (Brody, 1984, p. 88). In some sense, she thought, the metaparadigm needs justification. Given that the metaparadigm is supposed to be fundamental to the discipline, the lack of an argument for it is surprising. Second, Fawcett's discussion presupposes that scientific inquiry requires "rules" for identifying relevant problems and phenomena, research techniques, character of the data, methods of analysis, and so on (Fawcett, 1984, p. 85). What is remarkable is not the idea that such things are required by science, but that they needed to be identified *prior* to the conduct of research. This seems a bit paradoxical: before knowing anything about the objects of study, scientists have to determine what the objects are and how they might best be investigated.

While these two features of the discussion of nursing's metaparadigm are somewhat surprising, they make sense when understood against the background of the received view of theory. The idea of metaparadigm is a development of Kuhn's conception of a paradigm (Kuhn, [1962] 1970). While Chapter 16 will discuss Kuhn in some detail, one or two points will suffice here. A paradigm includes (among other things) a theory, some striking applications or exemplars, and methods. According to Kuhn, paradigms make "normal science" possible, and normal science includes most of what we usually take to be scientific research. Kuhn's conception of a scientific theory was very close to the received view. Indeed, *The Structure of Scientific Revolutions* was intellectually explosive because it drew unexpected consequences about scientific progress from shared ideas about theory. In particular, like other mid-century philosophers of science, Kuhn took the creation and testing of theory to be the central scientific activity. Like the positivists, he thought that concepts were defined by their place in theory, and that abstract theories determined the domain of a scientific enterprise. Kuhn's radical conclusion was that science was not progressive. Rather, paradigms changed during periods of revolution. Scientific revolutions were like gestalt shifts, and the adoption of a new paradigm meant the adoption of new theories, new concepts, and new methods. Fawcett's idea that inquiry requires "rules," and that these are (in a sense) prior to normal science is thus directly drawn from Kuhn, and it is part of what Kuhn shared with the received view.

What is a "metaparadigm"?

The word "metaparadigm" was introduced by Margret Masterman in her critique of Kuhn (Masterman, 1970). Masterman famously identified 21 senses of the term "paradigm" in Kuhn's book. She clustered these into three main groups, and she called the primary group "metaphysical paradigms or metaparadigms" (Masterman, 1970, p. 65). For Masterman, a metaparadigm was not a special kind of paradigm that was more general or abstract than an ordinary paradigm. When Fawcett and other nurse scholars adopted the term (e.g., Hardy, 1978), however, it became exactly that. Nursing's metaparadigm is the most abstract set of concepts and themes in the discipline, and it determines the proper domain of nursing inquiry. Under the umbrella of the metaparadigm, there are supposed to be several paradigms. Fawcett identified these with grand theories or conceptual models. Subsequently, others argued that there are qualitative and quantitative paradigms, totality and simultaneity paradigms, and so on. The metaparadigm serves to unify the various paradigms into a single nursing discipline.

Fawcett's metaparadigm thus unifies the discipline of nursing in precisely the way that mid-century philosophers of science thought a discipline should be unified: by its highest level concepts. It is thus no surprise that Fawcett did not try to justify or defend the metaparadigm. Unity, according to both Kuhn and proponents of the received view, is a top–down affair. There is no logic by which such unifying theories and concepts are discovered. They are stipulated, and their justification comes through the subsequent empirical testing of the theories. Given this view, it would make no sense to try to justify the metaparadigm. The best that could be done is exactly what Fawcett does: to survey existing work and try to find unifying concepts. The idea that nursing must have a metaparadigm is thus drawn from mid-century philosophy of science, and it relies on central ideas of the received view.

Levels of theory

The idea of a metaparadigm for nursing fits into a larger view of the shape of nursing science: there are different levels of nursing theory, and the levels are arranged in a hierarchy. Below the level of the metaparadigm, there are a number of grand theories (or conceptual models). Middle-range theories fall below the grand theories, and micro-range theories (sometimes called practice theories or situation-specific theories) fall below them. The earliest clear expression of this hierarchy is probably Jacox's essay "Theory construction in nursing: an overview" (1974), where she distinguished between middle-range and grand theory. Fawcett distinguished levels of theory as early as her essay "The relationship between theory and research: a double helix" (1978), and the idea of a hierarchy of nursing theories remained central to her work (Fawcett, 1984, [1985] 1999, 2005b; Fawcett & Alligood, 2005).

As we saw in Chapter 2, the rise of middle-range theory reinforced the idea that nursing theories formed a hierarchical structure, in spite of the fact that some early proponents intended to do away with grand theory entirely. Essays like Higgins and Moore's "Levels of theoretical thinking in nursing" (Higgins & Moore, 2000) confirm the continuing commitment to this idea. It is interesting to note that, prior to the 1970s, nurse scholars did not distinguish between grand and middle-range theory. The idea of theoretical levels was mostly promulgated by nurse scholars who were citing philosophers of science in the logical positivist tradition.[2]

The continuing influence of the received view can be seen in nursing discussions of how the levels are distinguished, how they are connected, and why they are regarded as necessary.

How the levels are distinguished

When nurse scholars discuss the levels of theory, they distinguish the levels in terms of abstraction and generality. Grand theories are "highly abstract theoretical systems that frame our disciplinary knowledge within the principles of nursing, and their concepts and propositions transcend specific events and patient populations" (Higgins & Moore, 2000, p. 180). Within the domain set by the concepts of the metaparadigm, grand theories propose broad generalizations. Middle-range theories, by contrast, are limited to particular patient populations or other circumstances. Microrange theories are further limited in their applicability. In this first respect, the levels of nursing theory clearly follow the dictates of the received view. The differences among the levels of nursing theory are directly analogous to the difference between, for example, the Newtonian theory of the tides (a middle-range theory) and the three fundamental laws of motion (the grand theory). On the received view, theories are distinguished by their level of generality, and the most general theories frame the knowledge of a discipline. Many nurse scholars hold exactly this view today.

How the levels are related

The relationship among the levels of theory also mirrors the received view. Understood as axioms, the fundamental laws of a theory are expressed in a theoretical vocabulary. As a result, they can entail no observable consequences by themselves. Less abstract laws have to be formulated by adding observable concepts and specific information about local domains. The resulting middle-range theories are more testable than grand theories because they entail specific, observable hypotheses. Moreover, testing a middle-range theory indirectly tests the grand theory from which it is derived. If the middle-range theory fails, its failure suggests that the grand theory is mistaken.

---

[2] Dickoff and James's view of theory is an exception. They articulated different levels of theory, but their way of identifying and relating the levels was not the same as the received view of theory. The idea of levels that became entrenched in nursing (e.g., Higgins & Moore, 2000) owes very little to Dickoff and James's work.

These dictates of the received view fit the way nurse scholars have described levels of nursing theory. Nurse scholars have argued that middle-range theory may be derived from grand theory (Liehr & Smith, 1999, p. 88; Fawcett, [1985] 1999, p. 6; Peterson, 2009, p. 31). Moreover, grand theories are tested through the middle-range theories associated with them:

> *"In essence, then, evaluation of the testability of a grand theory involves determining the middle-range theory-generating capacity of a grand theory. The criterion of testability is met when the grand theory has led to the generation of one or more middle-range theories."* (Fawcett, 2005b, p. 133)

Middle-range theories need not always be derived from grand theory. They may also be developed directly through research (Nolan & Grant, 1992; Liehr & Smith, 1999). However, many writers urge that such "inductively" developed middle-range theory must be ultimately tied to one grand theory or another (Cody, 1999; Fawcett, 2005b). This too follows the pattern of the received view. As we saw in the previous chapter, "experimental laws" may be discovered inductively, but the scientific project is not finished until these low-level regularities can be explained in more fundamental terms. Inductively derived middle-range theories would be composed of experimental laws or empirical generalizations, according to proponents of the received view.

Why the levels are supposed to be necessary

A robust tradition of middle-range theory development has resisted the idea that middle-range theories must be linked to grand theories (Nolan & Grant, 1992; Lenz *et al.*, 1995). This has led to some debate in the nursing literature. Perhaps the sharpest response to those who would divorce grand and middle-range theory has been William Cody's essay "Middle-range theories: do they foster the development of nursing science?" (Cody, 1999). Cody identifies three kinds of middle-range theory: those derived from grand theory, those invented independently by nurses, and those "borrowed with little or no alteration from another discipline" (Cody, 1999, p. 12). He argues that the last category should not be considered nursing science. "There are vast differences," he writes, "among the philosophical bases of schools of thought in medicine, physiotherapy, psychology, family science, nutrition, and pharmacotherapy, and differences among the philosophical roots of disciplines" (Cody, 1999, p. 11). Theories must be logically consistent with the concepts and philosophical assumptions of the discipline, and Cody supposes that these will be expressed by the most general theories. Therefore, if a middle-range theory is "rooted in a nonnursing paradigm, the likelihood that a logically consistent and semantically coherent theory rooted in nursing will emerge is nil" (Cody, 1999, p. 11). On pain of logical and conceptual incoherence, Cody argued, middle-range theories must be linked to the grand theories of a discipline.

Cody is an articulate and prolific proponent of the "simultaneity paradigm" in nursing, and he takes this paradigm to be opposed to both positivist and postpositivist philosophies of science. His arguments about middle-range and borrowed theory are important, and will be engaged below. For now, the point to be recognized is that the received view of theory continues to influence nursing scholarship, even among those who seek to distance themselves from logical positivism. Cody argued for the necessity of grand theory on the grounds of conceptual coherence and disciplinary integrity. The argument presupposes that the primary concepts of a discipline are carried by the most abstract theories, and that these grand theories determine the boundaries of the discipline. Moreover, disciplines are differentiated by their most general theories and concepts. Basic sciences are therefore distinct and conceptually independent. As we saw in the foregoing chapter, this is exactly what the received view said about theories and disciplines.

Borrowed theory

Cody's argument against divorcing middle-range theory from grand theory is also an argument against borrowing theory from other disciplines. We saw in Chapter 1 that the concern about borrowed theory and its place within the discipline of nursing is as old as nursing research. In the 1950s and 1960s, however, the questions were framed differently than they are now.

In Johnson's essay "The Nature of a Science of Nursing" (1959b), she did not contrast borrowed with unique theory. She assumed that different fields (both within and outside of health care) will share theories, concepts, and goals. She was concerned with a different problem, one that was discussed throughout the 1960s: How are nurses to select, evaluate, and modify theories that already exist? Johnson emphasized the role of nursing's social mandate in the selection of theories from other disciplines:

"The major determinant in the selection of knowledge from the basic and applied sciences pertinent to nursing is nursing's specific and unique professional goal. It is proposed here that the body of knowledge called the science of nursing consists of a synthesis, reorganization, or extension of concepts drawn from the basic and other applied sciences which in their reformulation tend to become 'new' concepts. It is further proposed that these 'new' concepts will be concerned largely but not exclusively with the causation, character, and process of the tension growing out of stress and disturbing internal or interpersonal equilibrium, or both. They will lead to the development of theories of nursing intervention which will yield predictable (and desirable) responses in patients when implemented in nursing care." (Johnson, 1959b, p. 292)

In Chapters 1 and 2, we saw how these concerns were debated within the nursing literature. Notice, however, that Cody's worry about conceptual incoherence does not appear. Borrowed concepts and theories were thought to need reformulation, but not because of any purported conflict with a metaparadigm or grand theory. The pressure to reformulate concepts came from the bottom up, not the top down. Johnson is suggesting that concepts and theories should be modified to create better descriptions of the causal systems that nurses needed to manipulate in their interventions. A similar view about borrowed theory was defended by Walker (1971,

p. 430), and it continues to be endorsed in recent editions of her textbook on theory construction (Walker & Avant, [1983] 2005).

The idea that borrowing concepts from other disciplines would cause conceptual incoherence arose in the 1970s. John Phillips, for example, argued strongly against borrowed theory on grounds that anticipate Cody's argument. He opened his essay "Nursing systems and nursing models" with the remark:

> *"Since the primary goal of nursing theory is the generation of knowledge specific to nursing, the process of theory building must be couched in a nursing frame of reference. Otherwise, the obtained knowledge will not be nursing knowledge which can be used to build or expand nursing science or be used for nursing education, practice, or research."* (Phillips, 1977, p. 4)

In the essay, Phillips articulated four models of health on which nurses have drawn, and he argued that each is inconsistent with the fundamental commitments of nursing. Only models that have been developed within nursing—he mentions Rogers' life process model and Johnson's behavioral systems model—can provide the basis for nursing knowledge. This concern with conceptual models was manifested as early as Riehl and Roy's *Conceptual Models for Nursing Practice* (1974), and was developed in Fawcett's early work (Fawcett, 1980a, 1989).[3] Conceptual models were taken to determine the semantic space for theory development. It follows that borrowed theory is something alien and dangerous. It can be used only if it is tamed by subsuming its concepts within the scope of nursing's conceptual models. The idea that borrowed theory threatens conceptual incoherence therefore depends on the idea that the most abstract theories (conceptual models) fully define the basic concepts to be used in a discipline. Here again, we encounter echoes of the received view of theory.

Conclusion: the relevance gap and the philosophy of science

The relevance gap between theory and practice was first identified by Conant in the late 1960s (Conant, 1967a, 1967b), but it was not widely recognized until the 1980s. When it began to be discussed, nurse scholars complained that the language of nursing theory was opaque and that the principles put forward had little to do with the interests of practicing nurses. Professional nurses did not feel that the knowledge produced by theorists responded to their needs. The historical discussion of Chapter 2 showed that the rise of the grand theory tradition in nursing coincided with the adoption of ideas from mid-century philosophy of science, and that the relevance gap between theory and practice opened as grand theory became influential.

---

[3] In this period, there was some disagreement about the relationship between conceptual models and grand theories; some held that they were distinct (e.g., Fawcett, 1980a), others assimilated them (e.g., Riehl & Roy, 1974). For now, we will assimilate them. In Chapter 15, we will look more closely at the idea of a conceptual model.

In this chapter, we have seen how specific philosophical ideas were incorporated into nursing metatheory. Having unpacked those philosophical ideas in Chapter 8, we are in a position to see how a relevance gap is a natural consequence of the received view of theory.

From the point of view of mid-century philosophers of science, scientific theories at the top levels were not supposed to be useful for solving practical problems. Abstract and general theories represented *pure* science. Indeed, it would only slightly overstate their view to say that a relevance gap was the mark of true science. The first way in which the received view pushed open the relevance gap, then, is through the interpretation of "theory" and "science." Science is the activity that develops theories, and proper scientific theories are pure. Nurse scholars similarly identified theory with the development of a basic science. Fundamental theories in the science of nursing, on this view, *should not* be relevant to practice. Knowledge relevant to practice, according to the received view, would have to be developed by applied nursing science. The needs of a profession would be met by middle-range and micro-range theories. The relevance gap, then, would be a temporary phenomenon. It takes time to develop basic theories and to derive the applications from them. While there may be a relevance gap now, further development of middle-range and micro-range theories will close it.

The sharp division between theories and values promoted by mid-century philosophers of science served to further exacerbate the problem. After practice theory lost its influence, nurse scholars adopted the idea that the values of the profession should be reflected in indirect ways. The values and social mandate of the profession influenced the metaparadigm concepts and themes. The professional values of nursing thus did no more than circumscribe the pure science of nursing. Professional nursing's need for knowledge that would help solve specific problems was not reflected in the disciplinary structure.

Mid-century philosophy of science thus framed a view of nursing science where a relevance gap between theory and practice was natural, if not inevitable. Nursing science was basic, and nursing theories did not have to be applicable to professional problems. Relevant micro-range theory would have to wait on the development of nursing grand and middle-range theories, and nursing values were to have no direct influence on the research enterprise. It is no wonder that the knowledge produced by such an enterprise seems irrelevant to practitioners.

If the view of science promoted by the nursing consensus of the 1970s were the only or best way to think about science, then we would have to accept the existence of a relevance gap. But we can and should expect nursing research to serve the needs of professional nurses. In Part II, we began to turn the consensus view of the nursing discipline upside down. We saw that it was possible to think about nursing science as fundamentally responsive to the values of nursing. Philosophers of science have shown that the philosophical ideas about theory that were incorporated into the 1970s consensus can be overthrown too. The next steps toward closing the relevance gap, then, are to understand why the received view was criticized and rejected in philosophy, and to see how those objections affect nursing conceptions of science.

Rejecting the received view

The received view of theory suggests a particular image of the sciences. Understood as an axiomatic system, a theory is structured like a pyramid. The fundamental laws (axioms) are at the apex. These entail a larger number of middle-range theories. The large body of observation statements is at the base, supporting the whole edifice. Since the theories in different sciences incorporate different fundamental laws, then they must remain separate. Each theory defines its own central concepts and stands on its own foundation of observation. The received view thus permits only two images of the scientific landscape. If science is unified, then it forms one great pyramid. This image treats science as a reductionist enterprise, where everything is ultimately explainable by the laws of physics. If science is not unified, then the scientific landscape is a city of pyramids, each standing on its own observational foundation and crowned with its own grand theory. To think of science as a plurality of paradigms is to imagine it as many independent pyramids.

Informed by the received view of theory, nurse scholars have thought of their discipline as a pyramid distinct from the other pyramids in the health sciences neighborhood. Unified by the metaparadigm at the apex, a number of paradigms spread out below, each supported by its own middle-range theories. This image encodes a number of key ideas that have been criticized by philosophers of science: that there are levels of theory, that distinct theories have unique concepts, that theories are independently supported by observation, and that there is a theory–observation distinction. This chapter will work through the philosophical arguments against these ideas. By understanding why philosophers of science stopped thinking about science in this way, we can begin to more deeply appreciate the contributions of postpositivist philosophy of science to nursing.

Holistic confirmation

The necessity of auxiliary hypotheses

According to the received view, theory testing is a matter of deriving observable statements (hypotheses) from the statements of the theory. If the hypothesis is observed to be false, then as a matter of logic, at least one proposition of the theory must be false. Many philosophers of science also held that if the hypothesis was observed to be true, then (under the right conditions) it supported the theory. The received view entails that separate theories are supported by distinct bodies of observation. Two theories at the same level define different concepts and have distinct laws. This is true of both the most abstract theories and of middle-range theories. Hypotheses are statements couched in the observational language, and they are deduced (with the help of bridge laws) from the theory. Because each theory has a distinct set of observational consequences, their empirical successes or failures are independent. As the metaphor of the pyramids suggests, a theory is supported by those theories and observations directly below it in the hierarchy. Theories at the same level (or in a different pyramid entirely) are confirmed or disconfirmed independently. This idea was famously challenged in Willard Van Orman Quine's "Two dogmas of empiricism" (Quine, [1953] 1961). Somewhat later, Hilary Putnam articulated a more elaborate version of the argument (Putnam, 1974).

Putnam pointed out that even the most straightforward deduction of a hypothesis from a theory required the support of additional assumptions. Putnam used the discovery of a new planet as an example. Uranus was discovered by telescopic observation in the late eighteenth century. Newton had already shown how to derive the orbit of a planet from his laws of motion, and had done so for the known planets. So, when Uranus was first observed, astronomers set about deriving its orbit. To their surprise, they found that the predicted orbit of Uranus did not match its observed orbit. According to the received view of theory, this ought to be a clear case of disconfirmation. Deducing Uranus' orbit from Newton's laws is a purely mathematical matter. The position of Uranus in the night sky is observable, and the prediction was shown to be false. Therefore, Newton's laws of motion should have been rejected or modified. Surprisingly, the astronomers did neither. They immediately postulated that there must be another, as yet unobserved, planet that was causing the deviation of Uranus' orbit from its predicted path. The planet subsequently known as Neptune was observed just where the astronomers predicted. These astronomers responded to the failed prediction about Uranus' position in exactly the opposite of the way prescribed by the received view. Even so, it was an important scientific success. What happened?

Putnam drew several important lessons from this episode. First, any derivation of a prediction from a theory requires "auxiliary hypotheses." These add information and are necessary for the derivation, but they are not part of the theory. In the case of the discovery of Neptune, the initial calculations supposed that there were only seven planets. This presupposition is in no way part of Newton's theory. As far as the theory was concerned, there could be any number of planets in our solar system. Similarly, the derivation presupposes that the planets move through a vacuum with no resistance. Without auxiliary hypotheses such as these, no observable consequences at all would follow from a theory (Putnam, 1974, p. 225).

A second important insight is that theories are not rejected—and should not be rejected—simply because they have false observational consequences. Any prediction from a theory will make some kinds of simplifying assumptions (e.g., that friction can be discounted). Such assumptions make the calculations easier, but they also mean that the predictions will be inaccurate. Theories should be rejected, Putnam suggested, when there is an available alternative. In the early nineteenth century, there was no viable alternative to Newton's theory. So, when the predictions failed, scientists held onto Newton's theory and looked among the auxiliary hypotheses for the source of the error (Putnam, 1974, p. 227). Neptune was discovered because astronomers rejected the auxiliary hypothesis that there were only seven planets.

Auxiliary hypotheses and borrowed theory

Auxiliary hypotheses do not always take the form of simplifying assumptions. Sometimes they are substantive results from other disciplines. Consider, for example, the development of the germ theory of disease. Early nineteenth century medicine was still dominated by the ancient Galenic theory. On this view, diseases are the result of imbalances of four humors (blood, phlegm, black bile, and yellow bile). Proponents of the germ theory proposed, instead, that small particles invaded the body and caused disease. By the early nineteenth century, microscopes had identified a whole world of small objects. The germ theory predicted that persons who suffer from the same disease would be infected by the same germs. John Snow was an early proponent of the germ theory. He became famous for removing the handle of the Broad Street pump and pioneering the methods of epidemiology. He also used microscopes. When Snow was investigating the London cholera outbreak of 1854, he tried to use microscopic techniques to identify the germs that might cause the disease. He failed to find what he was looking for. Just as the deviations in the orbit of Uranus might have been taken to refute Newton, the failure to identify the germ that caused cholera might have been taken as a refutation of the germ theory. Snow did not despair. He concluded that his microscope had simply failed to find the germs. Snow's research into the germ theory of disease thus presupposed a large body of knowledge about microscopes. Ultimately, 30 years later, the cholera bacterium was identified microscopically. But why suppose that the later microscopic observations were reliable when the earlier ones were not? Why not refuse to accept the results of any observations made with a microscope, just as Galileo's critics refused to look through his telescope? The answer is that microscopes are constructed with the aid of theories that have been independently tested. The explanation of how a microscope works and why it is reliable depends on theories of optics.[1] In this way, testing a theory can depend on ideas drawn from very different domains.

If these reflections are correct, then it is a mistake to think that a theory is supported only by those theories and observations below it in the theoretical hierarchy. Confirmation of scientific theories is "holistic" in the sense that a theory might get support from theories at any level of abstraction or generality. What matters is not the level or the domain for which the theory was designed, but the substantive content of the ideas. Snow's account of the cholera epidemic helped support the germ theory of disease because it showed that the contagion flowed from a single source. In turn, as the germ theory was supported from other quarters and by other methods, it supported Snow's account of the epidemic. There are no principled limits on where one might look to find auxiliary hypotheses that will help support (or undermine) a theory. Empirical support does not flow from the base to the apex of the theoretical pyramid. Indeed, these arguments show that there are no pyramids at all.

Consequences for nursing

These arguments against the received view have profound consequences for the way in which nurse scholars have thought about science. As we have seen, nursing discussion of borrowed theory and middle-range theory changed during the 1970s. Prior to this time, nurse scholars thought that borrowed theory would probably need to be modified to accommodate the new nursing phenomena. During the 1970s, nurses became concerned with the uniqueness of nursing theory. Nursing theory was supposed to develop its own resources, not rely on the results of other disciplines. The arguments in this chapter show that this stance toward borrowed theory serves to *weaken* nursing scholarship, not strengthen it. When a scientist draws on a theory that has been confirmed in another domain, she adds the empirical support of that domain to her view.

For example, the theory of planned behavior has often been used by nurse scholars. This theory was developed in social psychology (Ajzen, 1985), and some have worried that it is not a genuine nursing theory (Villarruel *et al.*, 2001). To insist, however, that it be reformulated in novel nursing terms would be to cut off the support available from existing tests in a variety of domains. The theory would be made unique to nursing at the cost of its empirical validity. Moreover, reformulating existing theories so that they fit the "hermeneutic context" of nursing grand theories (cf. Cody, 1999, p. 11) is an exercise that makes sense only if science is envisioned as a city of pyramids. The arguments we have seen so far show that theories and disciplines should not be conceived as independent. Sharing theory with other disciplines will strengthen nursing knowledge, not dilute it.

---

[1] The story is more complicated. Hacking (1983) has an excellent discussion of microscopy. One of its consequences is that our confidence in the reliability of microscopes does not rely entirely on theoretical considerations. Practical manipulations play a crucial role.

Failure of the theory–observation distinction

A keystone of the received view of theories is that theoretical concepts are distinct from observational concepts. Mid-century philosophers of science took this idea over from empiricism. On an empiricist view, observational knowledge is unproblematic. I know—with certainty, in a direct and immediate way—that I see a white patch or taste something sour. The problem of epistemology is to show how this kind of observational knowledge can justify knowledge of something unobservable. In science, the interesting and powerful theories postulate a host of unobservable entities. But how can the mechanisms of viral reproduction be known when they are too small to observe? Hence, the main epistemological questions for mid-century philosophers of science concerned the justification of theory. And as we have seen, the answers they developed presupposed a strict theory–observation distinction. The whole enterprise of logical positivism, and the ensuing philosophy of science, rested on the idea that observation was distinct from theory. In the 1950s and 1960s, philosophers of science began to call the theory–observation distinction into question.

The vagueness of the distinction

A first problem with the dichotomy between theoretical and observational concepts is that the distinction is vague. There is no clear line between what is observed and what is postulated as a theoretical entity. Imagine looking out of an open window at a tree (cf. Maxwell, 1962). This seems to be a clear case of "observing the tree." Imagine now that the window is closed. The light passes through the glass, but this does not mean that the tree is not observed. You are still observing the tree. Now, remember that you are wearing glasses. The glasses refract the light to "correct" your vision, and without your glasses you cannot see the tree. This case is not so happy: Do you see the tree, or just an image of the tree? Now suppose you are looking through binoculars, or a low-powered telescope, or a high-powered reflector telescope, or a digital telescopic camera, or an X-ray telescope. These devices produce images, but some are highly processed. At one end of this continuum, there is a simple and unproblematic observation of a tree. At the other end, there is the use of an instrument to detect the effects of an entity that is not itself observed. At what point do concepts become "theoretical" and in need of special justification?

The distinction between what is observable and unobservable is not just vague, it seems arbitrary. The difference depends on accidents of human physiology. After all, if our eyes responded to lower wavelengths, we would "see" temperature in the way we see color. As humans happen to be constructed, we perceive color and temperature with different sensory modalities. The received view of theory depends on a clear difference between theory and observation, but there does not seem to be any principled way of making it clear.

The role of training

Another kind of problem with the observation–theory distinction was raised independently by Norwood Hanson (1958) and Michael Polanyi (1958). These authors pointed out that, in the sciences, observation is a skill to be learned. Hanson imagined a vacuum tube viewed by a physicist:

> At school, the physicist had gazed at this glass-and-metal instrument. Returning now, after years in university and research, his eye lights upon the same object once again. Does he see the same thing now as he did then? Now he sees the instrument in terms of electrical circuit theory, thermodynamic theory, the theories of metal and glass structure, thermionic emission, optical transmission, refraction, diffraction, atomic theory, quantum theory, and special relativity (Hanson, 1958, pp. 15–16).

Of course, there is some sense in which anyone who viewed the object would see the "same" thing. But only the physicist (trained during a time when vacuum tubes were common tools of research) would *see* the glass-and-metal object *as* a vacuum tube.

Kuhn argued for the same idea and used the example of Sir William Herschel's discovery of Uranus in 1781 (Kuhn, [1962] 1970, p. 115ff). During the eighteenth century, Kuhn contended, at least 17 astronomers observed a "star" that was probably Uranus. None saw a planet because, at the time, astronomical theory held that there were only six planets. Herschel made observations with an improved telescope, and he noticed that the object was larger than ordinary stars. When he detected that the object was moving, Herschel concluded that he was seeing a *comet*. Like his predecessors, his observations were influenced by the theory. Since there were exactly six planets and many comets, a moving object must be a new comet. Calculating the object's orbit, Herschel failed to fit the orbit into a normal cometary path. After several months of trying, Herschel and his colleagues decided that the object must be a seventh planet. This was an important, if small, change in astronomical theory. The number of planets was no longer fixed, so it was possible that there were more to see. And indeed, in the first decades of the eighteenth century, over 20 new planetary objects (asteroids) were identified. The change in theory (not just telescope technology) allowed astronomers to see celestial objects in new ways.

Observation takes training, and training is shot through with theory. Once the point is seen, examples are easy to multiply. Much clinical research depends on a particular diagnosis, and this is heavily influenced by existing theories of disease. Or again, a good interviewer knows how to ask questions that lead to interesting answers. An interviewer who knows the subject's social and cultural background will be able to ask much better questions than one who is naïve. In these and many other cases, the background information (both theoretical and practical) influences *what* and *how* things are observed. Most observations in science could not be made at all without training in the relevant theories and techniques. This result is a problem for the received view because it took observation to have a special epistemic role. Observation needed to be theory-neutral because it was the means of deciding among theories. If observation is always theory-laden, then theory testing cannot proceed in the way that proponents of the received view thought it did.

Observation and theory testing

The argument that observation is theory-laden generates a new problem for the philosophy of science. Not only must the received view of theory be wrong about theory testing, it is not clear that scientific theories can be legitimately tested at all. If observation depends on theory, and the theory is supported by those very observations, then the justification is circular. The observations justify the theory and the theory justifies the observations. This problem is a significant starting point for postpositivist philosophy of science. There are two responses that indicate the way out of this circle. First, the arguments above show that the difference between observation and theory is a matter of degree. Some statements are more observational (and less theoretical) than others. In theory testing, the description of the evidence should not bias the test against any of the theories that are being tested. For example, in a study that tries to adjudicate between the theory of planned behavior and a social cognitive theory (cf. Dzewaltowski *et al.*, 1990), one would need observations that are not biased toward one or the other theory. Fortunately, this is not difficult because most descriptions of behavior are neutral between these two theories. It is therefore possible to design a test that would speak for one theory and against the other, even if all observations are theory-laden to some degree. This shows that observation may be neutral without being absolutely free from theory.

Another way out of the apparently circularity created by theory-laden observation is to note that the theory informing the observation is distinct from (and supported on different grounds from) the theory being tested. One of the ways in which observation becomes theory-laden is that a theory is used to create a technology that produces the observations. The theory explains why the technology is reliable, and it helps interpret the output. The observations made with the aid of the technology are thus the product (in part) of the theory. To interpret the observations made with a microscope as evidence of bacteria, for example, requires a theory about how the instrument is reacting to the environment. But theory being tested is not about light waves; it is about bacteria. If the theories are very different, and they are supported by distinct bodies of evidence, then the justification is not circular (Wylie, 2002). Here, we make contact with the earlier point about holistic confirmation: a theory is more strongly supported when it can be related to theories in other domains.

Levels of theory and interdisciplinary research

The idea that there are levels of theory is deeply embedded in the received view, and is a crucial part of many nurse scholars' image of the discipline. To see why this aspect of the received view was rejected by philosophers of science, let us return to an example that was used to illustrate the received view in Chapter 8: the gas laws.

Theory change and level mixing

The ideal gas law says that pressure (p), volume (v), and temperature (t) have a constant relation (n and R denote constants that are different for distinct gases):

$$pv = nRt$$

This means that changing the pressure of a gas while keeping the volume constant will change the temperature. This regularity is exhibited when a bicycle tire gets warmer as it is filled with air. The volume stays constant (more or less), but the pressure increases, hence the temperature must increase. Or again, the lid on a sealed container of warmed leftovers will depress as they cool; lower temperature correlates with lower pressure. This empirical regularity was discovered in the seventeenth century. In the eighteenth century, physicists found that if they treated a gas as composed of tiny particles that bounced elastically off the walls of the container (and each other), they could mathematically derive the ideal gas law from Newton's laws of motion. This "kinetic theory of gases" thus explained the ideal gas law.

From a positivist point of view, this episode in the history of science seems simple enough. Pressure, temperature, and volume are straightforwardly observable and measurable. The ideal gas law is expressed in the observational vocabulary, and it captures a regular relationship among these observable quantities. The kinetic theory of gases postulates unobserved, theoretical entities—molecules of gas—and shows how the observable regularity can be deduced from laws expressed in a theoretical vocabulary. The observed relationship among pressure, temperature, and volume is thus explained by a deeper theory. The observed regularity of the ideal gas law, in turn, serves to confirm the kinetic theory of gases, providing its observational justification.

While the ideal gas law looks like it nicely fits the received view of theory, matters are not so simple. Pressure, volume, and temperature are supposed to be observational, according to the positivists, because we can sense them directly. A change in pressure or temperature can be felt by hand. So, measuring devices such as thermometers or pressure gauges simply quantify and make more precise something that can be directly experienced. Given the strict theory–observation distinction, this experiential meaning is the content of the concepts of temperature, pressure, and volume. Wilfred Sellars pointed out that once the kinetic theory is devised, things change in a deep way (Sellars, 1963). A gas is no longer conceived as a homogenous, continuous substance; it is a huge number of little particles flying around in space. Temperature is the energy that the little particles have—the faster the particles move, the higher the temperature. To feel the pressure of a warm breeze is to feel the molecules in the air striking your face and imparting their energy to your skin. The concepts of temperature and pressure no longer have a merely experiential meaning. Scientific research changes our conception of what observable things *are*.

Similar examples can be found across the sciences. In medicine, prior to the germ theory of disease, fevers were a category of disease. The Galenic theory of disease held that a fever was a class of diseases caused by an excess of "hot" humors (blood and yellow bile). After the germ theory was accepted, a fever was no longer a kind of disease. Elevated body temperature is now understood as part of the body's repertoire of immune responses. Fever is thus a symptom of the underlying disease. In this way the germ theory of disease changes what it is to have a fever. Sellars' point is another argument against a strict theory–observation dichotomy, but it also undercuts the idea that theories form a hierarchy (the "levels picture" as Sellars calls it). On the received view, generalizations about fevers (how long they last, how they can be reduced, etc.) would be couched in the observation language. If the germ theory was to be a proper scientific theory, generalizations about fevers would have to be deduced from the germ theory, and thereby explained. But not only are no deductions forthcoming, they could not be constructed. The germ theory changes the concept of a fever. The old (pre-germ theory) generalizations about fever are thus not explained at all because the old generalizations are replaced by new ones. The levels picture thus fundamentally misrepresents the important change that occurs when one theory replaces another.

Theoretical integration

The levels picture also misrepresents the way in which scientific theories are integrated. As an example, consider (again) John Snow's work on cholera. Snow is celebrated as one of the founders of epidemiology. Prior to the nineteenth century, the dominant explanation for epidemic disease outbreaks appealed to miasmas, which were conceived as similar to a poison gas or "bad air." This explanation fit with the Galenic theory, since some diseases were already understood as bad airs produced in the body by the humors.

Proponents of the germ theory of disease, like Snow, sought a different explanation of epidemics. During the 1854 London cholera epidemic, Snow interviewed residents to determine which households suffered the disease. He found that many of the victims drank water from the Broad Street pump. Plotting the incidences on a map, he showed a pattern that clustered around the pump. As a result of Snow's research, drinking water was identified as the source of the disease.

In his work, Snow pioneered some of the basic methods of epidemiology. It is important to notice that the evidence and the theory are cast in population-level terms. While Snow favored the germ theory over the miasma theory, scientists and physicians as yet had no biological explanation of the epidemic. They knew that the water—rather than the air—was the source of the disease, but they did not yet know why. Thirty years later, when microscope technology and technique had improved, the cholera bacterium was identified. The germ theory of disease substantially supported the growing science of epidemiology by providing a mechanism that explained the patterns identified through maps, statistical analysis, and other methods.

According to the received view, the germ theory of disease and Snow's theory of epidemics would be theories at different levels. Appeal to germs as the cause of disease explains other aspects of disease than their distribution, while Snow's epidemiology primarily explained population-level phenomena. This makes Snow's theory of epidemics a middle-range theory under the grand theory of disease. But this is an inaccurate depiction of their relationship. First, the epistemic support between the two theories is mutual, not unidirectional. On the received view, testing lower-level theories serves to test (and thereby support) theories that are higher, but higher-level theories do not support lower levels. By contrast, the success of the germ theory provided substantial support to epidemiological explanations by providing the underlying mechanisms. And, as we saw, support for germ theory through microscopy indirectly supported epidemiological explanations. Moreover, the concepts of epidemiology are not defined by the concepts of germ theory plus some additional, local information. The concept of the "environment," for example, is crucial to epidemiology, but not part of germ theory. The germ theory of disease is therefore not a theory higher up in the same theoretical pyramid as Snow's theory of epidemics. Forcing these theories into a hierarchy obscures their deeper integration.

Consequences for nursing

Consider again Phillips' (1977) contention that there are different models of health care, and that nursing must develop a unique model if it wants to build a knowledge base for nursing practice. Phillips' root idea is shared with the received view: unique high-level concepts (conceptual models) are necessary to distinguish scientific domains. This results in the city-of-pyramids vision of the scientific landscape. But such a vision makes it impossible for disciplines to communicate, to share models, concepts, or explanations, or to develop models that bring together elements of different disciplines. As the example of epidemiology shows, the investigation of complex phenomena makes progress when scientific projects that employ different concepts and methods can be linked together in a nonreductive way.

The failure to make sense of more complicated examples of interdisciplinary research was especially important to philosophers of science who were interested in the life sciences. If we attend to the recent history of these disciplines, it is quite clear that progress has been made by building models that span domains. The possibility of much productive interdisciplinary research thus requires a different philosophical understanding of science (Bechtel, 1986). Because nursing phenomena are multidimensional, with biological, psychological, and social aspects, this argument is one of the most important reasons why nurse scholars should reject the received view and conceptualizations of their discipline that mirror it.

Conclusion: rejecting the received view of nursing science

The received view of theory was an important account of science. It influenced many of the scientific disciplines that arose during the twentieth century. When nursing assimilated these ideas in the 1970s, they were common enough to be common sense. But philosophy of science is a dynamic field, and by the 1970s a critical mass of philosophical argument had accumulated. This chapter has discussed three of the reasons why philosophers moved away from the received view.

Fundamentally, the received view misrepresents scientific practice. Its picture of hypothesis testing obscures the ways in which theories support each other. Borrowing theory is a powerful and pervasive scientific strategy, but on the received view it is difficult to see how different theories could be combined. The received view also tried to draw a strict theory–observation distinction. A strict distinction is untenable, and it misrepresents the profound ways in which research can produce conceptual change, even for observables. Finally, the idea that theory must fit within a hierarchy of levels distorts the way in which theories work together to provide scientific understanding. Much scientific progress has been achieved when theories from different domains are integrated. When philosophers turned their attention to complicated examples—the kinds of phenomena that concern nurse scholars—they found that the levels picture made the science impossible to understand. The notion that science is a hierarchy of axiomatic theories must, therefore, be abandoned.

Chapter 9 argued that several central ideas of the received view are embedded within nursing metatheory. Even those who reject logical positivism rely on its main ideas to frame the discussion. Nurse scholars in the phenomenological tradition defend their position as a distinct paradigm within the disciplinary metaparadigm. Quantitative researchers who embrace postpositivism conceptualize their work with the hierarchy of grand, middle-range, and micro-range theories. And while the theory–observation dichotomy has been roundly rejected, nurse scholars have not exploited the way that mechanistic, biological models help reconceptualize the phenomena of health. The roots of the received view run deep in nursing discourse. Unearthing them will require a fundamental rethinking of the idea of a nursing science.

Part IV
The Idea of a Nursing Science

Introduction to Part IV

In spite of its rejection by philosophers of science, the received view continues to influence contemporary debates about nursing theory and research. The discussion so far has concerned two issues: value-freedom and the structure of theory. In Part II, we saw how the idea that science must be value-free was an important part of the arguments that brought down practice theory. Chapter 5 argued against scientific value-freedom and Chapters 6 and 7 developed the idea that a fundamental evaluative commitment—the nursing standpoint—should drive nursing research and theory development. Part III addressed the conceptions of theory structure in nursing. While many nurse scholars have abandoned the received view, Chapter 9 showed that key concepts of the received view continue to influence the nursing debate. Chapter 10 reviewed the reasons why philosophers of science rejected the received view of theory. The conclusions of Part III tell us how *not* to think about the structure of scientific theories. But how then *are* theories structured? How are different theories—whether at the same level or different levels of generality—related to each other? This part will begin to develop a positive account of nursing science.

Questions about theory structure have special significance in the nursing context. A concern with unity has inspired much reflection in nursing: What unifies the discipline and makes nursing knowledge unique? Grand theory and the metaparadigm remain important to nurse scholars because they provide a clear account of unity and uniqueness. It is commonly thought that nursing needs grand theories, conceptual models, and the metaparadigm because without them, the discipline has no unity. The critical arguments in Chapter 10 undermine the philosophical foundation for this understanding of nursing knowledge. The idea of a nursing standpoint, developed in Chapters 6 and 7, goes some way toward rebuilding that foundation. The capacity of the nursing discipline to create unique knowledge about human health is based on the professional nurse's perspective on patient care. Nursing knowledge arises from the commitments to the value and betterment of nursing, as well as the real problems of human health encountered in nursing practice. The unity and distinctness of the discipline is thus grounded by professional practice.

While the nursing standpoint provides a starting point for thinking about the unity and distinctness of nursing, it does not address all of the concerns. When writing about middle-range theory, William Cody argued against the picture that has been emerging in the previous chapters. He rhetorically asked:

"Are the scholars who are working in the middle range on myriad topics in this way, then, really developing nursing science or merely elaborating the vast patchwork quilt of applied-science nursing, which admits of any topic remotely related to any portion of the entire discipline?" (Cody, 1999, p. 11)

Cody was arguing that middle-range theory development should not proceed without reference to grand theories. The concern is that, if nursing theories are developed in response to the problems of professional nursing without guidance from grand theories, then nursing research becomes a fragmented enterprise. Nurse researchers would do little more than fix limited problems with practical scope. If this were true, nursing would be an applied science. It could not reach its aspiration to become a scholarly discipline. This picture of nursing is unsatisfactory, but not just because it is unflattering. It fails to do justice to the results that nurse researchers have already achieved. The results of Parts II and III thus raise pointed questions about the structure of theory and the unity of the nursing discipline, and the goal of Parts IV and V is to address them.

What would nursing knowledge look like if it were not structured in terms of grand and middle-range theory? One important answer to that question arises from the work of Afaf Meleis and Eun-Ok Im. They have promoted the idea of "situation-specific theory" as the appropriate form for nursing theories. In some ways, situation-specific theories neatly fit the demands created by the critical chapters above. Situation-specific theories are directly responsive to the problems of professional nurses, and they encompass the values of professional nursing. Chapter 11 will present Meleis and Im's situation-specific theories and evaluate them in the light of some examples of successful nursing research. While they are an advance on earlier views, Chapter 11 will argue that situation-specific theories are not fully adequate as an account of the structure of nursing theory. Their limitations can be traced to lingering influences of the received view in nursing. Chapter 12 will present an alternative shorn of those influences. It depicts theories as coherent sets of propositions, where coherence is generated by the relationship of questions to answers. Theoretical propositions are answers to questions about human problems or striking phenomena. These answers raise further questions, and the aim of scientific theorizing is to answer these questions in a systematic way. As we will see, this is a view of theory that fits both the natural and the social sciences. It therefore does not differentiate between theories developed with qualitative methods and those developed with quantitative methods, a point that will be important in Part VI.

Some of the most powerful research in the health sciences build models that cross domains. Understanding biology at the molecular level, for example, explains disease mechanisms and has resulted in many new therapies. Many of the treatments of modern medicine have been made possible because we have scientific theories about how the large-scale, morphological features of humans (including psychological as well as physiological features) relate to their organs and tissues, the cellular structures of the organs and tissues, and ultimately the molecular and genetic machinery of those cells. Nursing has resisted this kind of model building on the grounds that it is reductionist. It seems to violate the value that professional nurses put on the whole person. At the same time, there are many examples of nursing research that construct, develop, or apply causal models. Chapter 13 will work through this dilemma, arguing that while nursing's commitment to the whole person is important, it does not preclude nursing research that investigates the micromechanisms of human health.

Postnursing theory inquiry

Passion for substance

In 2008, Afaf Meleis gave a lecture to the *Combined 12th International Philosophy of Nursing Conference and 15th New England Nursing Knowledge Conference* with the paradoxical title "Theoretical Foundation for Nursing Science: Post-Nursing Theory." To those who had followed her trajectory since the 1980s, declaring an era of postnursing theory was a logical extension of her work. In 1987, while other metatheorists were engaged in fierce debates about the character of the nursing discipline, Meleis called for nurse scholars to go beyond the philosophical dichotomies and focus on developing the substance of their field (Meleis, 1987). Subsequently, she has portrayed grand theory, middle-range theory, and micro-range theory as a historical progression, wherein the discipline moved from discipline-framing theories toward the concrete and practical (Im & Meleis, 1999). In Meleis' view, a "postnursing theory" form of inquiry would not eschew scientific theorizing. Rather, nurse scholars should turn their attention away from arguments about metaparadigm concepts or developing new grand theories, and focus on the practical needs of nursing.

Meleis' vision of nursing inquiry encompasses several points that have been supported by the arguments of the foregoing chapters. In her view, nursing inquiry must be politically and morally engaged. In her well-known essay, "ReVisions in knowledge development: a passion for substance" (1987), she discussed the alliance between feminism and nursing. Feminism, she argued, can contribute both a methodological orientation and a domain of substantive concern. She generalized the specific concern for women and women's health by calling for "gender-sensitive knowledge," which would consider "the sex of the researcher, the sex of the subject, and the context of the research encounter" (Meleis, 1987, p. 11). The research questions asked from this perspective highlight the importance of nurse and client experience, perception, and meaning. Meleis was thus an early proponent of the idea—defended in Chapters 6 and 7—that the moral and political commitments implicit in the nursing profession should set the agenda for disciplinary research. In subsequent essays, she deepened this commitment (Meleis, 1992, 1998; Meleis & Im, 1998). In a 1992 essay, she identified one of the characteristics of the nursing discipline as "its mission to develop theories to empower nurses, to empower the discipline, and to empower clients" (Meleis, 1992, p. 113). The empowerment she envisioned included attention to nursing services and institutions as well as systematic research into nursing problems. The passion for substance, therefore, was not just a call for more research with practical relevance. It was an attempt to reorient the nursing discipline from a top-down emphasis on the metaparadigm and grand theory to a bottom-up structure that began with a commitment to the profession. Meleis' passion for substance, then, fits the critique of nursing theory that was developed in Parts II and III.

Situation-specific theories

In the late 1990s, Meleis and her colleague Eun-Ok Im began to promote "situation-specific theories" as a way of bridging the relevance gap (Im & Meleis, 1999; Meleis, 1998):

> *"Situation-specific theories [are] theories that focus on specific nursing phenomena that reflect clinical practice and that are limited to specific populations or to particular fields of practice. Situation-specific theories are put in social and historical context and they are not developed to transcend time, a socially constraining structure, or a politically limiting situation. They are theories that are more clinically specific, that reflect a particular context, and that may include blueprints for action. We propose that situation-specific theories could be the discipline of nursing."* (Im & Meleis, 1999, pp. 13–14)

Im and Meleis frame situation-specific theories as the most concrete forms of nursing inquiry. The definition thus intentionally reflects a contrast between situation-specific theories and grand or middle-range theories. Im and Meleis are philosophically and methodologically pluralistic about situation-specific theories, arguing that they are consistent with a variety of epistemological, ontological, and evaluative assumptions (Im & Meleis, 1999; Im, 2005). They emphasize theories that describe the responses of narrowly defined groups of patients, such as menopausal Korean immigrant women or female clerical workers in the United States (Im & Meleis, 1999, p. 18). However, they do not limit situation-specific theories to the characterization of patient experiences. Some research might aim to explain "the linkage between the observables such as vital signs and laboratory findings and the unobservables, and between those normal and abnormal physiologic and psychological processes, which suggest causal factors and subsequent treatment" (Im & Meleis, 1999, p. 15). Im and Meleis thus attempt to bridge the relevance gap by promoting theories with direct clinical relevance, which might take the form of either understanding patient experience or explaining the underlying mechanisms.

While Im and Meleis do not trace the genealogy of situation-specific theory all the way back to the practice theorists of the 1960s, there is an important sense in which situation-specific theory is their descendent.[1] Both emphasize clinical relevance and a commitment to professional values. As developed by Ellis (1968, 1969) and Conant (1967a, 1967b), practice theory was to remain close to the specific concerns of practitioners. Because the goal was to develop prescriptions for nursing practice, not just descriptions or explanations, practice theory incorporated the goals and values of professional practice. However, by the time Meleis wrote the "ReVisions" essay, the consensus of the 1970s had taken hold. Most nurse scholars saw the discipline as governed by the metaparadigm and grand theories. The dispute was over the relative merits of qualitative and quantitative paradigms. The new philosophical landscape made situation-specific theory different from 1960s practice theory in at least two ways. First, situation-specific theory emphasizes patient experience and perception in ways that the earlier practice theorists did not. Situation-specific theory thus uses the resources of qualitative research that were developed in the 1980s. Second, it presupposes that nursing inquiry proceeds at different levels of abstraction. Situation-specific theory is defined in contrast to grand and middle-range theories (Im & Meleis, 1999, p. 17). While it has the same fundamental orientation toward the discipline as practice theory, then, the debates of the 1970s and 1980s give situation-specific theory a distinct character.

Postnursing theory inquiry

Meleis has argued for some time that the future of the nursing discipline will be to grow away from nursing-specific theories and toward a discipline that is integrated into the health sciences:

> "As nurses and societies become comfortable with the uniqueness of what nurses can offer, knowledge for nursing will then be knowledge for health care in general. It will be knowledge developed and utilized collaboratively by members of a number of disciplines. Therefore, nursing theories will become theories for health care, developed by nurses, physicians, occupational therapists, and others. There will no longer be nursing theories. There will be theories about health care, some of which are developed by nurses." (Meleis, 1992, p. 115)

Making a contribution to knowledge of health is a common aspiration for the nursing discipline; it is, after all, among Donaldson and Crowley's themes (Donaldson & Crowley, 1978). Meleis' remarks here are striking because she envisions a nursing discipline that is not isolated by adherence to a unique metaparadigm. What is the place of situation-specific theory in this picture? One might suggest that situation-specific theories are the substance of the discipline in the post-theory era. This seems to be the view expressed by Im and Meleis when they

---

[1] Im has called situation-specific theory a kind of practice theory (Im, 2005), but she does not use "practice theory" in Wald and Leonard's sense.

say: "We propose that situation-specific theories could be the discipline of nursing" (Im & Meleis, 1999, p. 14). Situation-specific theory seems to fit the philosophical framework being developed in this work. Should we take situation-specific theory to be the appropriate form for future nursing science?

One way to test whether situation-specific theories are the appropriate form for scientific research in the postnursing theory era is to look at some examples. Other health science disciplines recognize and use nursing research results. Does existing nursing research that has contributed to the larger understanding of health fit the criteria for situation-specific theory? A useful set of examples have been documented by Donaldson. Her essay "Breakthroughs in scientific research: the discipline of nursing 1960–1999" (2000), identified many cases of nursing research with broad significance. She defined a "breakthrough" as "knowledge that transcends its discipline of origin, in this case nursing" (Donaldson, 2000, p. 248). The criteria that she used to identify a breakthrough were (1) "the contribution was primarily to the discipline of nursing," but at the same time, (2) it "changed the prevailing thinking about a human health phenomenon" in another discipline, and (3) that the scholars in the other discipline acknowledged that nursing was the source of the new view (Donaldson, 2000, pp. 248–249).

Donaldson identified almost 60 breakthroughs in 11 research areas: person and family health, pain management, neonatal and young child development, research utilization, dementia care, site transitional care, health and violence, women's health, stress urinary incontinence, psychobiological health, and biobehavioral health. A striking feature of Donaldson's review is that they *fail* to fit the standard models for nursing research. With one exception, the studies were done without reference to nursing grand theory or conceptual models. High level, abstract theory did little or nothing to guide these breakthroughs.[2] There is no clear preference for qualitative or quantitative methods, nor any apparent cleavage between qualitative and quantitative forms of nursing knowledge. Research canvassed by Donaldson used the full range of methods available, from interviews and focus groups to surveys, clinical trials, and laboratory experiments. Even philosophical arguments about the value of autonomy and dignity played a role. Donaldson's examples, therefore, look like an excellent testing ground for any view of nursing research and theory in the postnursing theory era. Let us consider some of Donaldson's cases and determine how well they fit the criteria for situation-specific theory.

Research example: mastectomy

Background

Because of the success of breast cancer awareness and support programs, it is hard for us to imagine the approach to radical mastectomy taken by both physicians

---

[2] Since this is consistent with the earlier finding in (Silva, 1986), it does not represent a change in nursing research.

and nurses in the 1950s. By this time, radical mastectomy was a well-established surgical procedure. The literature in nursing discussed the emotional and personal impact of the surgery, but it emphasized the physical and physiological aspects of care. Consider, for example, a pair of articles published back-to-back in *The American Journal of Nursing*. The first, written by a physician, urged self-examination and briefly described the surgical procedure. The final section of the essay, titled "Psychological implications of mastectomy," is entirely composed of two paragraphs:

> *"Most patients with breast cancer who fully understand the nature of their illness get along with minimum mental distress. The physician should, therefore, explain the exact meaning of the patient's diagnosis, the type of therapy he expects to follow to control her disease, and what results she may expect. A good deal of the patient's fear of the unknown may be removed by such a free and open discussion—especially if the discussion is held in the presence of a member of her immediate family and her nurse."*

> *"Whenever a physician fails to inform his patient and her family about such matters as plan of treatment and expected results, he places an undue burden upon the nurse; she is forced to supply evasive answers to their questions. Her answers to their questions concerning the proposed treatment and its probable results should in no way reflect any difference of opinion from that of the treating physician. If the nurse is unable to attend the conference between the physician and the patient and her family, she should ask the physician for a summary of the information he has given them."* (Popma, 1957, p. 1571)

The companion piece, written by a nurse, attends primarily to postsurgical care, including the patient's physical position after surgery, exercises, diet, and dressing. The tone of the essay is illustrated by the fact that a narcotic is recommended before the first dressing change to help the patient "relax and be less apprehensive" (Alexander, 1957, p. 1572). Her final section, titled "Preparing for Home," begins with the remarks:

> *"Throughout the patient's hospitalization, she will, at intervals, be concerned about how her family will accept her. This will happen regardless of the support and assurance the nurse and doctor have offered. Once the patient has learned to accept herself, however, and to realize that she is still the same person she was before surgery, then and only then, will her family accept her, because she will be, and is, the same person they knew and loved."* (Alexander, 1957, p. 1572)

In these essays, the patient is presented as a lone individual. She will have concerns about how she will be accepted by others, but these are to be allayed by providing medical information about the course of treatment and prostheses. There is a striking absence of the emotional trauma, challenges to self-image, or the need for social support that we now believe to be so important for breast cancer survivors.

Patient responses to radical mastectomy

In spite of the physician-oriented tone of the 1950s' literature on breast cancer, nurses were seen as having a special role:

> "Concern over the cosmetic defect involved in the loss of the breast, or fear that the function of the arm may be impaired also occasionally deter women from seeking treatment. It has been our experience that the nurse, with tact and gentleness and a greater understanding that comes from being a member of the same sex, is better able to help the patient resolve these problems than is the physician." (Sugarbaker & Wilfley, 1950, pp. 334–335)

Physical, psychological, and social consequences for the patient of any surgery were clearly within the nurse's range of responsibilities. The gender-specific character of radical mastectomy added an additional dimension to nurses' care and concern. Breast cancer, its detection and treatment, and the whole range of consequences for the patient were therefore squarely within the nursing domain as nursing research expanded in the 1950s and 1960s.

Jeanne Quint-Benoliel (*née* Quint) was an early participant in the University of California at Los Angeles' pioneering program to train nurses in scientific research. She began a project that changed the character of physicians' and nurses' responses to radical mastectomy—and breast cancer more generally—by focusing "on the viewpoint of the woman who experiences mastectomy" (Quint, 1963, p. 88). Quint-Benoliel used participant observation and interviews to study a group of 21 women who had undergone radical mastectomy. Her contact began during the patient's hospitalization and continued for a year. The result was a rich description of the woman's initial shock, emotional and social responses to the surgery, and her anxieties about the future.

It is clear from Quint-Benoliel's presentation that these dimensions of the patient's experience and the meaning of the surgery to them were important to the nurses, but at the same time, difficult to confront. Nurses recognized that women who had undergone the procedure needed to talk. But time pressure, the patients' own unreadiness to talk, and the nurse's sense of personal vulnerability made it difficult to reach out. Quint-Benoliel's qualitative research showed that there was a clear need for special support for these patients, and she took nurses to have an obligation to provide it:

> "It is no small thing to have a breast removed for cancer, and adjustment to living with the change comes slowly. Most surgeons cannot offer the kind of sustained support which these women want. Perhaps this is not the surgeon's job, for what can he know of what it is like to be a woman?"

> "For nurses to accept responsibility in this problem, however, they must be willing to forego the practice of saying, 'That's the doctor's responsibility,' and be willing to face a problem which offers no easy solutions." (Quint, 1963, p. 92)

That there was a need for such support is something that is recognizable from the nursing standpoint, but not easily seen from other health care positions. "Not all doctors saw purpose in the study" she wrote (Quint, 1962, p. 205). Quint-Benoliel brought to the study a commitment to the overall well-being of the patient, not just her survival, as well as a commitment to the value of a nursing response to the patient's needs. Other nurses shared these commitments, but by highlighting the need for more substantial nursing support, Quint-Benoliel's research showed how the commitments required deeper knowledge and stronger action.

As Donaldson documents the progress of her career, Quint-Benoliel developed this early study into a more systematic description of the ways in which patients adjust to major health transitions (McCorkle & Quint-Benoliel, 1983). She studied different patient populations, and ultimately generalized her findings to all persons with a terminal illness. Quint-Benoliel's contribution to our understanding of human health, then, is a general theory about the "dynamic process and time stages of adaptation of humans to life-threatening illness" (Donaldson, 2000, p. 252). This theory began as a situation-specific theory, but it made a contribution to the discipline of nursing and to general knowledge about health because, ultimately, it was not limited to a specific patient population. Nursing knowledge grew because Quint-Benoliel was not satisfied to understand only women who had undergone radical mastectomy. She wanted to know why a larger patient population responded to a terminal diagnosis in the way they did.

Research example: pain management

Background

Pain assessment and pain management are central to the professional nurse's domain. Nurses have done substantial research on pain, investigating both pain interventionsand more general questions. Donaldson identifies a three-phase breakthrough in this area, beginning with Jean Johnson's experimental research. In the late 1960s and early 1970s, when Johnson began her research, questions about the measurement of pain focused on the idea of a pain threshold. The pain threshold was conceived as the intensity of the stimulation necessary for perception. It had already been recognized that the perception of pain was influenced by psychological factors. A patient's pain threshold might rise or lower, depending on his or her emotional state, information about the stimulus, environmental distractions, and so on. These results about the variability of pain perception, along with a growing body of physiological work, had led Melzack and Wall to postulate the gate-control theory of pain (Melzack & Wall, 1965). This theory proposed that pain was the result of several neural systems, and that higher cognitive processes modulated pain response.

Against this background, theorists had begun to suspect that pain experience had two components, sensory and reactive (Johnson, 1973; Johnson & Rice, 1974). The sensory component was "the type and intensity of sensation" described by words such as "burning" or "sharp" (Johnson & Rice, 1974, p. 203). The reactive component characterized the distressing or bothersome dimension of pain. This distinction raised a number of research questions. Could the two components be manipulated separately? What kind of information or environmental control might reduce the emotional or psychological component of pain? The latter question was important from a nursing perspective because nurses could influence the information about, or emotional color of, a painful stimulus. Nursing interventions had already targeted these areas, and the 1960s research on pain promised some hope of placing these interventions on a sound footing.

Sensory and distress components of pain

Johnson entered the debate about the pain threshold and its measurement with a series of experiments (Johnson, 1973; Johnson & Rice, 1974). She hypothesized, against the background of the gate-control theory of pain, that the sensory and reactive components could be independently manipulated. In her initial experiments, all patients were subjected to the same painful stimulus—a blood pressure cuff inflated to 250 mm while the subject squeezed a hand dynamometer (Johnson, 1973; Johnson & Rice, 1974). To separately manipulate the reactive component of pain sensation, Johnson provided the subjects with different kinds of information. For example, in one experiment, the subjects were divided into four groups. In the first, the experimenter provided a false description of the sensations that would be felt during the experiment. In the second, the subjects were given an accurate and complete description of the sensations to be experienced. In the third, the subjects were given an accurate, but partial, description of the sensations. The final group received only a description of the procedure and no description of the sensations. Subjects were presented with two scales, one marked "sensation" and the other marked "distress," and they were asked to rate their experiences on these scales at various times during the experiment (Johnson & Rice, 1974, p. 205). In this experiment, and the others like it, she found that the different information conditions affected the distress ratings, but not the sensation ratings. In other words, the distress and sensation components of pain were to some degree independent.

Johnson's experiments also showed that the character of the information given to patients affected their level of distress. Patients who were given either false descriptions of the sensations to be expected or no description of sensations at all had reliably higher distress scores than those given accurate information. Interestingly, there was no significant difference between the full and partially accurate descriptions. This result, Johnson recognized, had direct consequences for nursing practice.Giving a patient a description of the procedure, as was often done, was less effective than accurately describing at least some of the sensations that would be experienced. And it was not necessary for the description to be complete; a partial, but accurate, description worked just as well as a complete one. In subsequent research, Johnson and her colleagues sought more realistic contexts for their study of pain management. She looked at the effects of providing sensory information to patients undergoing surgeries and a variety of painful or uncomfortable procedures (see the references in Johnson et al., 1978; McHugh et al., 1982). She also tried to tease apart the relative contribution of coping strategies and sensory information to patient outcomes (Johnson *et al.*, 1978).

Breakthrough research and situation-specific theory

Did the nurse researchers develop situation-specific theories in these two cases of breakthrough research? Im and Meleis identify six characteristics of situation-specific theory:

> *"(1) a lower level of abstraction, (2) reflection of specific nursing phenomenon, (3) context, (4) readily accessible connection to nursing research and practice, (5) reflection of diversities in nursing phenomena, and (6) limitation of generalization."* (Im & Meleis, 1999, p. 16)

All of the breakthrough research surveyed by Donaldson reflects specific nursing phenomena and it all has a connection to nursing practice. Pain management is obviously central to nursing concern. And while Quint-Benoliel's efforts to understand the experiences of radical mastectomy were not initially seen as important, her research demonstrated that it was. Both research projects had clear consequences for nursing practice.

Nonetheless, while they satisfy some of the criteria, neither of these examples qualifies as situation-specific theory. They are not restricted to a low level of abstraction, and they did not limit their generalizations to a specific population. Quint-Benoliel began with the kind of population that Im and Meleis envision as the subject of situation-specific theory: women who have undergone mastectomy. Her research led to a much richer understanding of women's responses to the diagnosis and treatment of breast cancer. This portion of Quint-Benoliel's work might qualify as situation-specific theory, but Quint-Benoliel did not stop there. She generalized this research and developed a theory about how humans respond to the diagnosis of life-threatening illness. This is no longer limited to a specific population. Johnson's research, by contrast, was never limited to a particular nursing context. Her studies concerned pain experience, which is a universal human health phenomenon. Neither Johnson's nor Quint-Benoliel's research programs fit the criteria for situation-specific theory, and the rest of Donaldson's breakthroughs fare similarly. This indicates that, in spite of the strengths of situation-specific theory, we should not think of it as the whole substance of the discipline.

The examples of breakthrough science in nursing discussed above do not qualify as situation-specific theories because they are not limited in generalization or abstraction. Specific examples aside, there is some reason to think that such a limitation on abstraction would not be a good idea for nursing. Limiting generalization and abstraction would preclude nurse scholars from developing the more powerful theories on which context-specific interventions or theories draw. For example, in her recent discussion of situation-specific theory development, Im provides examples of nurse scholars whose research meets the criteria for situation-specific theory (Im, 2005). While these nurse scholars work with specific populations, they draw on theories or models that are general and abstract, such as the health belief model, the theory of reasoned action, and research on social support. The theory of reasoned action, for instance, is a theory from social psychology that applies to the intentional action of any human. If situation-specific theories, as defined, were the whole of the discipline, then nursing scholarship would not be charged with developing theories as general as the theory of reasoned action. They could draw on such theories, but their development would not be part of the nursing discipline. Im's own examples, however, clearly show that such general knowledge is required to solve nursing problems. Moreover, nursing research develops these models in ways that makes them more useful for professional nurses. Limiting the scope of situation-specific theories, therefore, makes them incapable of meeting the needs of the nursing profession.

Im and Meleis do not discuss the above concerns, perhaps because they are thinking about situation-specific theories in the context of grand and middle-range theories. They seem to have an implicit, background commitment to a hierarchy of nursing theory. This commitment invites a conflation of the *level of abstraction or generality* with the *relevance to practice*—a conflation which is quite common in the literature. On the standard view, higher-level theories are more abstract, less directly testable, and less directly relevant to practice. The most useful theories, then, must be at the lowest levels of abstraction and generality. But this is not true, as Donaldson's breakthroughs demonstrate. Professionals of all kinds know that some theories are useful precisely because they are explanatory generalizations that work across the specifics of context. Professional relevance and generality are therefore independent: general knowledge can be directly relevant to nursing just as well as contextual knowledge. To achieve professional relevance, then, we need not limit nursing inquiry to concrete, context-specific investigations.

Conclusion: revisioning nursing theory

The situation-specific theories proposed by Im and Meleis cohere with the perspective developed in this work. They are responsive to the needs of the profession, embed professional values within nursing inquiry, and promise to develop robust models, theories, and descriptions of nursing phenomena. As Im and Meleis characterize them, however, situation-specific theories are limited in their level of abstraction and the degree to which they can generalize across contexts. While some nursing research fits these criteria, the examples of breakthrough research do not. Therefore, while some nursing research will be situation-specific, we should not think of all nursing research in these terms. The source of the limitations to situation-specific theory, this chapter has argued, is the background commitment to a hierarchical conception of theory. If we are to disengage situation-specific theories from the hierarchy of theory, then we will have to rethink some of its defining characteristics. The character of nursing theory needs to be even more radically revisioned.

The structure of theory

Some of the most prominent and useful nursing research does not fit the consensus view of nursing theory. The breakthrough research projects identified by Donaldson (2000) are not related to grand theories or conceptual models. They do not fit neatly into the hierarchy of grand, middle-range, and situation-specific theory. On the contrary, they span levels of generality, reaching from general phenomena of health to population-specific concerns. Moreover, the breakthroughs were not constrained by the nursing metaparadigm. These theorists were successful because they drew on non-nursing intellectual resources and engaged non-nursing intellectual debates. The failure of nursing philosophy to account for some of the most successful nursing research, combined with the critique of the underlying account of theory (Chapter 10), makes the question of theory structure vivid. How are the propositions of a theory connected together? How are different theories related?

The questions about theory structure have, so to speak, a horizontal and a vertical sense. Nursing theories need to respond to the problems of practice. Donaldson's examples of breakthroughs show that, even when theories are general and powerful, breakthrough nursing research arises from professional practice. The "vertical" sense of the question about theory structure is thus: How are the propositions of a theory related to nursing problems? What makes Johnson's work on pain a response to nursing phenomena in a way that non-nursing research and theory about pain are not? The "horizontal" question is about how different theories are related to each other. Nursing research needs to draw on theories from other disciplines, and nursing scholarship should contribute to the other health sciences. But then how are the propositions of different theories related?

Walls and webs

The critical arguments in Chapter 10 suggest a postpositivist account of theory structure that is germane to nursing. Positivism envisioned theories as like pyramids; a small number of general laws were supported by larger number of middle-range theories, and these were supported (via bridge laws) by an even larger number of observations. Except at the top, each level supports the levels above it, and each level of theory is supported by the levels below. Ultimately, the observations support everything. Two of the arguments from Chapter 10 help motivate an alternative. First, empirical support for a theory often comes from theories in distant places, not just theories at a lower level. For example, theories about the refraction of light justify our confidence in the reliability of microscopes, which are necessary for observations in biology. Theories about cells are thus indirectly supported by theories about light. Theories get support from other theories at the same level of generality, not just from the observations within their domain. The second argument was against the theory–observation distinction. On the received view, observations needed to be independent of the theories they supported. The argument for the theory-laden character of observation showed that observations in science depended on theory. These two arguments conclude that scientific disciplines cannot be a number of freestanding and independent pyramids.

In an important critique, Quine suggested the metaphor of a spider's web (Quine, [1953] 1961) as an alternative to positivist ways of thinking about theory. A web is anchored at the edges, and each node is supported from all sides. All of science—indeed, all of knowledge according to Quine—is a single web. At the edges are observations and toward the middle are our most general theories. The web metaphor captures insights from both of the critical arguments against the received view. Any one theory is supported by the theories around it; changes in one part of the web can have distant ramifications. Also, while observations have a special role in science, they can be indirectly supported by other theories. For a wall or a pyramid, all of the support works from the bottom up. Bricks on the bottom support those above them. As a result, if a part of the foundation fails, it will destroy that part of the wall above it. In a web, by contrast, support is distributed across the whole. Break one strand, and the stress is picked up by other strands. To think of science as like a web, rather than a wall (or pyramid), is thus to think of it as a system of propositions that are mutually supporting. Any one theory is a part of the system, supported by and providing support to those parts around it.

In epistemology, the difference between the wall metaphor and the web metaphor is the difference between a *foundational* theory of justification and a *coherence* theory of justification. On a foundationalist theory, reasons for belief are traced back to epistemological bedrock. On pain of regress, foundationalists have argued, all knowledge must be supported by something that does not itself need further justification. In an empiricist view, for example, observation provides the foundation for knowledge. Observation statements of the proper form (e.g., "It seems as if I see something red.") cannot be called into question or doubted. Since they are certain, they neither need nor can have further justification. The argument that observation is always theory-laden (Chapter 10) undermines foundationalist approaches to justification: there is no such indubitable foundation. The coherence theory of justification begins by rejecting the requirement that knowledge have a foundation of certain and indubitable beliefs. Coherence—the way in which the parts of a theory hang together—is sufficient for justification. According to a coherence account, a theory is justified if it is more coherent than any alternative. Like the strands in a web, elements of a coherent theory support each other.

Questions and answers

The metaphor of the web is attractive, but it is empty unless we can say what the "strands of the web" amount to, and what it means for the parts of the web to "hang together." One way of explaining the relationship among parts of a theory (or among theories) relies on the relationship between questions and answers. In life, we are beset with various kinds of problems: how to find food, maintain our relationships with others, or preserve our health. These problems give rise to questions, and the solution to our practical problems requires refining the questions and finding their answers. Human knowledge is composed of propositions that answer our questions. Of course, not all questions respond directly to practical needs. We might also ask why the sky is blue, or why bears hibernate. This sort of curiosity is the origin of science, but notice that theories about the atmosphere or ecological adaptation may ultimately have practical consequences as well. (Perhaps, centuries later, they contribute to a response to global warming.) Knowledge grows because answers to any given question will give rise to further questions.

Knowledge is thus a web of statements (or propositions), each of which is either the answer to a question or the basis (presupposition) of another question. At the edge of the web are simple descriptions, such as the observation that the patient is restless, is flushed, or has an elevated blood pressure. These play a role similar to the observation statements of an empiricist view. As starting points for inquiry, they anchor our theories to the world. Unlike traditional empiricism (and positivism), however, there is no presupposition that these observation statements are independent of theory or that they are incorrigible. Understood in terms of the logic of question and answer, the function of observation statements is to raise questions. *Why* do some pregnant women have an elevated blood pressure? Is the patient restless because he is uncomfortable, or because of preoperative anxiety? The answers to these questions will take the form of statements, and each answer will be a new node in the web.

Coherence and confirmation

Thinking about a theory as a web of questions and answers not only helps understand how propositions are structured into theories, it also shows how theories are supported by evidence. When we answer a question like "Why do people get fevers?" with a story about the body's response to infection, it is natural to say that the answer is an *explanation* of the fever. Indeed, some postpositivist philosophers of science have identified explanations with answers to why-questions (van Fraassen, 1980; Garfinkel, 1981; Risjord, 2000). The story about the body's response to infection is justified insofar it is the best answer to the question, that is, the best explanation. Of course, what makes the account of infection the best explanation is not just that it explains fevers. It should allow us to answer lots of other questions too. Moreover, the claims about infectious agents give rise to a host of new questions: How do these agents enter the body? By what mechanism does the body raise its internal temperature? The justification for a theory, on this view, gets stronger as it answers more questions and is the basis of questions that are themselves answered. These links make the theory, and the web of science as a whole, more *coherent*.

Notice that to say that a theory is coherent is to make an implicit comparison. A theory is justified if it is more coherent than the alternatives. The object of some research (often called "theory-testing research" in the nursing literature) is to produce new evidence. Experiments, correlation research, and qualitative studies generate material that needs explanation. If an existing theory cannot explain the new evidence, then it is relatively incoherent. A new account that explains both the new and the old evidence would be more coherent than the old theory. Theories change, on this view, so as to be coherent with new observations. Scholars and practitioners are justified in accepting a theory if it is the most coherent theory available.[1]

An account of theory structure in terms of questions and answers also shows how theories can support each other. Sometimes, theories raise questions that need answers from another domain. The example of the microscope, mentioned above, shows that intertheoretical support can be provided at the level of evidence and observation. When a microscope provides evidence for a biological theory, it is taken to be reliable under the conditions. Why is it reliable? If a different preparation were used with the same microscope, would it still be reliable? These are not questions that biology can answer. Their answers depend on what is known about the construction of the microscope and character of the preparation. In this kind of case, the biological theories supported by the microscopic observations are also supported by the other theories. The whole, which now includes all of the linked theories, is made more coherent. Similarly, when nursing researchers draw on theories from social psychology, education, or genetics, they are using these theories to answer questions that arose from nursing. Both "borrowed" theory and nursing breakthroughs used by other disciplines integrate nursing research into the larger web of science. Insofar as non-nursing theories are used to answer nursing questions, or nursing theories used to answer non-nursing questions, nursing research is made stronger.

Horizontal and vertical questions

At the outset of this chapter, we noted that the questions about theory structure had horizontal and vertical senses. Nursing theories need to respond to both the problems of professional practice (vertical) and relate to other theories (horizontal). An explanatory coherence view of theory structure shows how nursing theory does both. Nursing knowledge emerges from the professional role of nurses when nurses

[1] For a more detailed and logically rigorous account of explanatory coherence, see (Thagard, 1992) or (Risjord, 2000).

undertake the commitment to make their unique perspective explicit. The nursing standpoint requires nurse scholars to take the problems of practice seriously. On a coherence view, this means that the distinctive intellectual contributions of nursing research are answers to questions that arise from practice. As nursing theory develops, more general questions and answers will arise. Since professional nursing is concerned with human health, it will be natural for nursing theorists to draw on the knowledge of the other health sciences. According to a coherence view, such horizontal relationships add empirical support to nursing knowledge. Nursing theory is therefore exactly that body of knowledge that supports nursing practice.

Breakthrough research revisited

Two examples of breakthrough nursing research were used in Chapter 11 to argue that situation-specific theory is too narrow a characterization of nursing inquiry. What do those examples look like when viewed from the perspective of an explanatory coherence account of theory structure?

Radical mastectomy

Quint-Benoliel's research began from the nursing problem of caring for women who had undergone mastectomy. Nurses knew that such patients needed more than care for their physical wounds, but they did not know how to provide it. The fundamental practical question, then, is: What kind of emotional and psychological support do mastectomy patients need? Before answering this question, Quint-Benoliel had to answer another: What is the character of the mastectomy patients' experience? To answer this question, she used participant observation and interviews. These revealed patients with more complicated experiences and broader needs than had been apparent to practicing nurses. By bringing something implicit in nursing practice to light, she expanded the knowledge base of professional nursing.

Quint-Benoliel's research did not stop here. The fact that mastectomy patients had unmet emotional and social needs raised further questions. What kind of emotional and social support best prepared patients for the next phase of their lives? How do a patient's emotional and social support needs change as she moves through the diagnosis, surgery, and recovery stages? And how does a diagnosis of breast cancer differ from diagnoses of other terminal diseases? In response to these questions, Quint-Benoliel began to describe the dynamics of patient response. With Ruth McCorkle, she showed how patients with a variety of conditions showed a steady decline in mood disturbance, even while symptom distress remained constant (McCorkle & Quint-Benoliel, 1983). This showed that patients come to terms with all kinds of serious illnesses in similar ways. At this point, her results were quite general and interesting to researchers in other disciplines.

Quint-Benoliel's research trajectory began with questions that arose directly from the concerns of professional nurses. Notice that while there was an immediate practical problem (how to care for mastectomy patients), the true scope and character of that problem was not clear at first. Her early research answered the initial questions, and those answers made the next round of questions more profound. By thinking of her research in terms of the questions that it was trying to answer, we can see how her early work directly illuminated nursing practice. The question-and-answer model also shows how her later concerns for a more general patient population arose naturally from her earlier work. The explanatory coherence account of theory structure thus shows how research can be both a scientific contribution to general knowledge about human health and distinctive work within the nursing discipline.

Pain research

Johnson's work on pain also has its origin in a problem of professional nursing. Her research was different from Quint-Benoliel's insofar as her topic was already the subject of interdisciplinary scientific research. The fundamental practical question was: How can pain be mitigated by nursing intervention? The gate-control theory of pain seemed to have some resources for answering this question insofar as it suggested that the sensory and reactive components of pain were distinct. The first step, Johnson recognized, was to clarify the distinction:

> *"Before the two-component concept of the pain experience can be useful in the clinical assessment of pain, it must be demonstrated that people can differentiate between the two components and make separate judgments about their intensity."* (Johnson & Rice, 1974, p. 204)

Johnson's experiments did just this, thereby showing how nurses might mitigate a patient's pain experience in nonpharmacological ways. Johnson's experimental research thus drew on non-nursing research that addressed one of professional nursing's central problems.

Johnson's research has another dimension that is illuminated by the nursing standpoint. Johnson showed that *accurate* sensory information modulates a patient's pain experience. Patient autonomy is among the values that animate the nursing standpoint. In this period, health care was a very paternalistic enterprise. It was not standard practice to tell the patient the truth about his or her condition or about the impending procedure. Using the accuracy of sensory descriptions as her experimental manipulation was not an accident. Johnson's choice to study accurate and inaccurate information reveals an implicit goal of supporting and expanding the autonomy of the patient. It is a move in the argument over what and how much to tell the patient. While it is generally applicable and of broad interest to the health sciences, Johnson's research question fundamentally arises from the values implicit in professional nursing. The explanatory coherence view of theory structure, when combined with the nursing standpoint, thus shows how research can be animated by the values of professional nursing, even when it is developing theories borrowed from elsewhere.

Borrowed theory

Concern about how theories from other disciplines might be used in nursing research arose in the 1960s. In Chapter 1, we saw how the debate about whether nursing research might borrow theory was tied up with concerns about the uniqueness of nursing research and the boundaries of the discipline. In the 1970s, the understanding of borrowed theory was reformed around the conception of theory nurse scholars were developing. On that view, nursing needed its own, unique theories, and theories drawn from other disciplines were not really part of nursing science. This view continues to be expressed:

> *"research that generates or tests theories from other disciplines is not nursing research. Furthermore, findings of such research build the knowledge base of the other disciplines. Since most nursing research falls into this category, the premise is that we are using precious resources to build a knowledge base with strong roots in other disciplines."* (Barrett, 2002, p. 55)

It is rather striking to say that most research by nurses is not nursing research. The consensus view of theory makes the rationale for this paradoxical view clear. Barrett is probably referring to the large body of research that uses the resources of other disciplines to develop nursing interventions. Intervention research is the lowest level of the hierarchy of theory, according to the standard view in nursing. Since higher-level theories contain the laws and concepts that govern lower-level theories, the development of interventions should be a matter deriving practical consequences. Intervention research thus applies theory, and in doing so it both tests the higher-level theories and develops practical technologies. Given this picture, it is natural to think of intervention research which uses borrowed theory as developing another discipline's theory.

The idea that interventions based on borrowed theory is not really nursing research and theory development rests on the received view of theory. What does intervention research look like when we view it from the perspective of the nursing standpoint and an explanatory coherence account of theory structure?

Research example: pain intervention

Consider a recent study of pain management by Stacy Friesner *et al.* (2006). These investigators asked "whether relaxation exercises added to standard medical therapy would result in improved pain-management outcomes" (Friesner *et al.*, 2006, p. 269). The gate-control theory of pain forms the theoretical background to this question. If the felt intensity of pain depends on cognitive and affective processing, then (as Johnson's research showed) changing the cognitive or affective response to pain stimulus would reduce the patient's feeling of pain. Friesner *et al.* ask about relaxation, which is a specific manipulation of the patient's affective response to a situation. They tried to answer their question by studying pain responses among patients undergoing chest tube removal after coronary artery bypass surgery. This population was well suited to answer their question. The process is painful, even with standard pharmaceuticals, and it occurs predictably. And because it is predictable, the process raises considerable anxiety among patients. Hence, if relaxation is going to work, its effects should be visible in this population. Friesner *et al.* measured pain by having patients point to a standard 10-point scale before, immediately after, and 15 minutes after the procedure. All of the patients ($n = 40$) received pharmaceuticals, and half of the patients received instruction in deep breathing techniques. The patients were told to begin the deep breathing exercise 5 minutes before the chest tube removal procedure, to hold their breath during, and to continue deep breathing for as long as they chose afterwards. The result of the study was rather dramatic: patients who used deep breathing reported pain scores that were two points lower, on average, both during the procedure and afterwards (Friesner *et al.*, 2006, p. 274).

The standard textbooks on theory development in nursing would treat Friesner's study as a "theory-testing" research. In this kind of study, a hypothesis is supposed to be derived from the theory, and the truth or falsity of the hypothesis then confirms or disconfirms the theory. Notice, however, that Friesner's study does not fit this model in some important ways. To see why, suppose their hypothesis that relaxation improves pain outcome had not been supported. On the positivist model of theory structure, such a result would falsify the theory. What theory would be falsified in this case? The gate-control theory does not seem to be in any danger. As a theory about the neurological and psychological processing of pain, gate-control theory makes no specific recommendations for behavioral interventions. Hence, the hypothesis may be false while the theory is true. This shows that the hypothesis about relaxation is not logically *derived* from the gate-control theory at all.

Friesner's research does test a theory, but it does not test the gate-control theory. The study is set up to test the hypothesis that relaxation exercises would result in improved pain-management outcomes (Friesner *et al.*, 2006, p. 269). The "theory" in this case is the intervention. If the evidence had shown no difference between control and experimental groups, it would have demonstrated that deep breathing exercises were not an effective way of controlling pain. It is worth noting that this test does follow a falsificationist line; most experiments do. An explanatory coherence view of theory does not reject falsificationism. It embeds falsification in a different context. An experiment like Friesner's produces new data to be explained. Data inconsistent with the hypothesis need explanation. One available explanation is that some element of the theory is false. An alternative explanation might be that the experiment was flawed. When a researcher is deciding how to handle a negative experimental result, the question is one of coherence. She has to determine which explanation is the most plausible in the light of the rest of her knowledge. The right choice will be the one that answers the most questions.

Borrowed theory and the nursing standpoint

Friesner's research does not test the gate-control theory of pain. Therefore, it is a mistake to think that this kind of research is testing theories from another discipline. There are, nonetheless, important connections between Friesner's research and the gate-control theory. A coherence view can illuminate the connections because it does not insist on a deductive structure for theory. From the perspective of the gate-control theory, research like Friesner's answers the question of *how* cognitive and affective responses can be manipulated. Johnson's research showed that description alone can change the distressing component of pain. Friesner's research is different because it is less cognitive. The intervention is not talk, it is action. Because Friesner's and Johnson's research programs answer questions that arise from the gate-control theory, they increase its coherence. In this sense, Friesner and Johnson were both developing the gate-control theory, even if Friesner's research was not testing it directly.

From the nursing standpoint, the questions look somewhat different. Friesner's project, like Johnson's, arises from the problem of pain management. Relaxation is a technique that is within both the nurse's and the patient's control. It is therefore the kind of intervention that both promotes nursing action and enhances patient autonomy. However, prior to this research, why think that relaxation would reduce pain experience? The gate-control theory provides an answer: if the neural processing of pain is modulated by other psychological or emotional factors, and these can be controlled through relaxation exercises, then relaxation ought to modulate pain experience. Friesner's questions thus make sense in the light of the theory because the theory explains why the intervention would be plausible. Once we free ourselves from the idea that explanations are always deductive, we can see this relationship in its proper light. The gate-control theory provides a context within which Friesner's intervention makes sense. Since the intervention was successful, the gate-control theory provides a plausible account of why the intervention works. And conversely, Friesner's intervention strengthens the gate-control theory by increasing the coherence of our overall understanding of pain and pain management.

Conclusion: piecing the quilt

The introduction to this Part introduced the concern that without grand theories to guide research, the discipline might become a "vast patchwork quilt" of borrowed theories and interventions (Cody, 1999, p. 11). This concern arises from a perspective that regards disciplines as independent. Each has its own concepts, theories, and methods. Borrowing is difficult, on this view, if not impossible. Part III showed how this view relied on the received view of theory, and it presented arguments against it. This chapter presented a different view about how theories are structured. It has embraced the quilt, and argued that the strength of nursing lies in its capacity to make connections and bridge differences. Theories are coherent sets of propositions, and they are made coherent by a question-and-answer structure. Each proposition of a theory is either the answer to a question or the presupposition (topic) of another. A theory should be adopted when it is the most coherent theory available, and one theory is more coherent than another when it leaves fewer questions unanswered.

Coherence is enhanced when theories from one domain answer questions raised in another. This means that a theory that connects with work in another discipline is more strongly supported than a theory that is unique to the discipline. It is crucial, then, for all disciplines to look at the work being done outside of their borders. If nursing's theories cannot be related to theories in medicine, biology, sociology, education, and so on, then nursing is weaker for it (and so are the other disciplines). Insofar as the pieces of the quilt can be sewn together, the whole is epistemologically stronger. Answering the questions of another discipline is therefore not a weakness of nursing, but a strength; and the links are reinforced as other disciplines can answer questions that arise out of nursing research.

No discipline owns a theory. The whole of science is a vast patchwork quilt of theories, and some of the most exciting leaps forward occur in those areas where the patches overlap and a number of theories are integrated into a rich, multidimensional understanding. Nursing lies in one of these areas of overlap, and the fundamental value of promoting and supporting the work of professional nurses blends all of those projects into a single enterprise. The domain of nursing science is the science that makes explicit the nursing standpoint.

Models, mechanisms, and middle-range theory

What is middle-range theory?

The enthusiastic literature on middle-range theory hides an ambiguity. Proponents blamed the relevance gap on grand theories, arguing that they

> "*were somewhat distant from the world of nursing practice and were neither developed from nor tested through research. Nursing theory as a type of knowledge in that era [the late 1960s to early 1980s] was often considered by both practitioners and researchers to be too abstract to be useful. As others have noted, nurses seemed to believe that to be theory, the knowledge needed to be obscure and lack immediate use and meaning. Therefore, theory was relegated to a place separate from research knowledge and practice knowledge.*" (Blegen & Tripp-Reimer, 1997, p. 38)

To close the gap, proponents of middle-range theory sought to develop theory that was more immediately useful, concrete, and meaningful to practitioners. Two conceptions of "middle-range theory" were put forward to satisfy this need. The dominant tradition sees middle-range theory as a level within a hierarchy of theories (Fawcett, 1978, 1984; Phillips, 1996; Liehr & Smith, 1999; Higgins & Moore, 2000; Fawcett & Alligood, 2005; Parse, 2005; Peterson, 2009). On this conception, middle-range theories are defined by contrast with grand and micro-range theory. They are more testable and applicable than grand theory, yet more generalizable than micro-range theory. Conceived in this way, middle-range theory fills the relevance gap by bridging the distance between grand theory and nursing practice. Chapter 9 showed how this understanding of middle-range theory depends on the received view.

The alternative way of conceptualizing middle-range theory arose from the critique of the received view. Suppe was among the philosophers of science who developed new ways to think about scientific theory. In Suppe's collaboration with nurse scholars, he proposed middle-range theory as a successor to the tradition of grand theorizing. Middle-range theory was meant to replace, not supplement, grand theory (Suppe & Jacox, 1985; Suppe, 1993; Lenz *et al.*, 1995). The relevance gap is closed by thinking differently about nursing science.

If we accept the philosophical critique of the received view (Chapter 10), then we need to take a closer look at Suppe's conception of middle-range theory. The "semantic conception of theories," of which Suppe was a prominent proponent, emphasized the use of modeling, especially causal modeling, in scientific understanding. In the philosophy of science, this view has helped illuminate the way that underlying mechanisms explain complex phenomena. While nurse scholars have not thought about their work in these terms, we will see below that some nursing research neatly fits this framework. However, it also raises an important concern. Nurse scholars have shied away from postulating causal mechanisms—or even borrowing research that does so—on the grounds that it is "reductionist." Since the early 1960s (if not before), nurse scholars have affirmed the value of holism. They have argued that nursing phenomena must be understood in their full complexity. An analysis of the parts (neurological mechanisms, social–psychological models, etc.) cannot support nursing knowledge. These arguments will be discussed and evaluated at the end of the chapter.

An old, new definition of middle-range theory

Perhaps the most misunderstood essay in the nursing literature is "Collaborative development of middle-range theories: toward a theory of unpleasant symptoms" by Elizabeth Lenz, Frederick Suppe, Audrey Gift, Linda Pugh, and Renee Miligan (Lenz *et al.*, 1995). This essay is routinely cited as the origin of the middle-range theory movement. They define middle-range theories in this passage:

> "[I]t is possible to divorce Merton's middle-range versus grand theory distinction from its positivistic underpinnings by recasting the definition of middle-range theories as follows: Theory and observation (experiment) use the same descriptive vocabularies. It is possible to distinguish those theories that postulate relationships between the (quantitative or objectively coded qualitative) values of those descriptors and those that do not. A time-relativistic distinction can be drawn between those descriptive terms that can currently be measured or objectively coded and those that cannot. Hence, at time t, a theory T is middle range if it postulates relationships between the (quantitative or objectively coded qualitative) values of its descriptors and if it is possible to measure or objectively code those descriptors. Thus, whether a given theoretical formulation can be considered middle range depends on the adequacy of its empirical foundations and is not simply a matter of its scope or level of abstraction." (Lenz et al., 1995, p. 3)

Notice how Lenz *et al.* distance their definition from a hierarchical conception of theory. It has become common to characterize middle-range theories in terms of abstraction, generality, and testability. These criteria distinguish middle-range from grand theory by its place in the theoretical hierarchy. But notice that at the end of the passage, Lenz *et al.* conclude that whether a theory is "middle-range" does *not* depend on its scope or level of abstraction. Their view of middle-range theory is therefore quite different from the common understanding. Lenz, Suppe, and their collaborators were recommending that nursing science focus on the development of substantive models of phenomena relevant to nursing. In retrospect, calling these models "middle-range theories" was a tactical error. It permitted their work to be assimilated to the existing philosophical framework, rather than appreciated as a radical transformation of nursing science.

A reader tuned to the philosophical debates of the 1980s and 1990s will recognize the strong influence of Suppe on this paragraph. Suppe was among the philosophers who proposed the semantic conception of theories as a successor to the received view (van Fraassen, 1980; Cartwright, 1983; Giere, 1988; Suppe, 1989). They argued that the received view had overemphasized the form or syntax of theory. This led earlier philosophers of science to treat theories as axiomatic systems, and as we saw in Chapter 10, this led to all kinds of philosophical trouble. In contrast, the proponents of the semantic conception wanted to focus on what theories were about, on their content (semantics) rather than their form (syntax). In recent work, many philosophers of science have turned away from theories entirely and toward models and mechanisms as the elements of scientific knowledge.[1]

The semantic conception and the received view

To illustrate the difference between the received view and the semantic conception of theory, consider again the ideal gas law and the kinetic theory of gases. The ideal gas law postulates a relationship among temperature, pressure, and volume, roughly $pv = t$. According to the received view of theories, this relationship was understood as a law. Indeed, it was an "experimental law" since it does no more than describe a relationship among observable properties. The kinetic theory of gasses treats a gas as a cloud of particles. The particles have mass and momentum (hence kinetic energy), and their behavior is described by Newtonian mechanics. "Particles" and their properties are theoretical concepts, according to the received view. They cannot be observed. On the received view, therefore, the kinetic theory of gases is understood as a more general theory, and the ideal gas law is derived from the laws of the kinetic theory. The kinetic theory is thereby made more testable because the derivation relates the theoretical concepts of particle mass and kinetic energy to the observables of pressure, temperature, and volume.

We saw in Chapter 10 that one reason why the received view is unsatisfactory is that it misrepresents the relationships among theories. When the kinetic theory of gasses is introduced, it changes the meaning of "pressure" and "temperature." Because pressure and temperature are reconceived in terms dictated by the kinetic theory, theoretical concepts influence the observational concepts. In the quotation above, Lenz *et al.* preface their new definition of middle-range theory with this very

---

[1] This Chapter follows Giere's lead in assimilating the 1980s literature on the semantic conception into recent work on models and mechanisms (Giere, 2000).

point: "theory and observation (experiment) use the same descriptive vocabularies" (Lenz *et al.*, 1995, p. 3). After the kinetic theory is introduced, pressure and volume are no longer mere observable properties. Temperature becomes the mean kinetic energy of the particles, and pressure becomes the transfer of kinetic energy to the walls of the container. An increase in temperature means that the particles have more kinetic energy; they move faster. If the volume is constant, faster moving particles will collide with the walls of the container more often, thereby increasing the pressure. After the kinetic theory of gasses is introduced, the ideal gas law changes its character. There are not two systems of laws with different vocabularies; there is a single model of gases with a single vocabulary.

When Lenz *et al.* say, therefore, that a theory is middle-range "if it postulates relationships between the ... values of its descriptors and if it is possible to measure or objectively code those descriptors" (Lenz *et al.*, 1995, p. 3), the "descriptors" must be different from the observation vocabulary of the received view. In the kinetic theory, the values of the descriptors must include the particles' mass and momentum (not the pressure, temperature, and volume of the gas). If so, then the "relationships" between the "descriptors" are nothing more than specifications of how these elements interact: particles of the gas collide with each other and the container walls, and when they do, they transfer energy. (Of course, the kinetic theory uses Newton's laws to say this with mathematical precision.)

In their definition of middle-range theory, Lenz *et al.* require that the descriptors be measurable, and they introduce a puzzling "time-relativistic distinction" between theories with measurable and unmeasurable descriptors. What they mean is this. At a particular time, suppose scientists do not know how to measure the mass or momentum of a gas molecule. As long as the descriptors are not measurable, the theory is not middle-range. At a later time, suppose they discover a way to measure the mass and momentum of gas molecules. When they do, the model changes from a speculative idea to a testable, middle-range theory. This is why Lenz *et al.* say that "whether a given theoretical formulation can be considered middle-range depends on the adequacy of its empirical foundations" (Lenz *et al.*, 1995, p. 3). The ability to measure the descriptors makes the model testable, hence a proper middle-range theory.

Middle-range theories as theoretical models

In his own work, Suppe used the idea of a "physical system" to capture what was distinctive about the semantic conception of theories:

> "The notion of a physical system *provides us with a convenient starting point for sketching and motivating this alternative [to the received view]. A science does not deal with phenomena in all of their complexity; rather, it is concerned with certain kinds of phenomena only insofar as their behavior is determined by, or characteristic of, a small number of parameters abstracted from the phenomena.... A physical system for classical particle mechanics is concerned with the behavior of isolated systems*

of extensionless point-masses which interact in a vacuum, where the behavior of these point-masses depends only their positions and momenta at a given time. . . . Physical systems, then, are highly abstract and idealized replicas of phenomena, being characterizations of how the phenomena would have *behaved* had *the idealized conditions been met."* (Suppe, 1989, p. 65)

What Suppe describes in this passage has been called a "model" by other philosophers of science. The semantic view of theories treats scientific theories as models (or more precisely, a class of models). To distinguish them from the "conceptual models" often discussed in nursing, and to highlight their scientific character, let us call them "theoretical models" (cf. Giere *et al.*, 2006).[2]

Theoretical models, as Suppe indicates, always treat an idealized and isolated part of the overall phenomenon. They are idealized in the sense that they pick out some properties or objects and knowingly ignore others—in the way that the kinetic theory treats gas molecules as perfectly elastic and without shape or size. Theoretical models also isolate the systems by ignoring known influences. In these ways, theoretical models are artificial constructs. They are known to be inaccurate precisely because they idealize and isolate the system. Of course, all maps and scale models are artificial constructs too. Like maps and scale models, a theoretical model identifies a small part of the overall phenomenon. Precision is sought for specific aspects of the phenomenon—just as some maps precisely represent topography while others precisely represent political relationships. Throughout the history of science, and across disciplines, theoretical model building has been a fruitful mode of inquiry.

Physical and nonphysical theoretical models

Many middle-range theories used by nurses are theoretical models. The theory of planned behavior (Ajzen, 1985), for example, postulates that an intentional action may be analyzed into a number of elements: behavioral beliefs, attitudes toward the behavior, normative beliefs, a subjective norm, perceived behavioral control, and so on. The theory proposes a relationship among these: roughly that the strength of the behavioral intention is the sum of the strengths of the attitude toward behavior, the social norm, and the perceived behavioral control. The theory of planned behavior is thus a model in just the same sense as the kinetic theory of gasses is a model. An important difference is that the kinetic theory proposes physical elements, while the theory of planned behavior proposes psychological elements: beliefs, thoughts, and attitudes. This shows that a theoretical model need not have physical entities as its elements.

Psychological models ignore outside influences just as physical models do. Human agents get tired or drunk, and when they do, the theory of planned behavior will poorly represent their actions. Similarly, the theory of planned behavior

---

[2] What Reed and Lawrence call "clinical conceptual frameworks" are theoretical models, as that term will be used here (Reed & Lawrence, 2008).

ignores the emotional dimensions of cognition and their influence on intention. Like other models, then, the theory of planned behavior idealizes and isolates a system. Theoretical models typically sacrifice some scope or depth, but they gain precision. While they do not answer all of our questions about a phenomenon, they do answer many of them. Indeed, it is only with models of this kind that we can explain *how* something works.

The challenge of precision in nursing models

The theory of unpleasant symptoms (Lenz *et al.*, 1995, 1997) illustrates a further feature of models and their use in nursing. Lenz *et al.* wanted to model the way in which unpleasant symptoms interact. They analyzed the symptom experience into three primary elements: antecedent factors, symptoms, and performance. Each of the main elements is further analyzed. Symptoms have distress, duration, intensity, and quality dimensions. The antecedent factors may be physiological, psychological, or situational. As further developed in (Lenz *et al.*, 1997), they postulated that the three main elements acted through a feedback loop. Antecedent factors influence the symptom dimensions. Multiple symptoms influence each other, and the symptoms influence performance. The patient's performance (which includes daily activities, social interaction, and cognitive abilities) then feeds back, influencing both the symptom dimensions and the antecedent factors. In the first presentation of the model, they said that "it cannot yet be considered a true middle-range theory" (Lenz *et al.*, 1995, p. 9). This was because they did not have good ways to measure the elements (descriptors). The primary progress documented in the update (Lenz *et al.*, 1997) was the development of various assessment tools. This made it possible to begin testing and using the theory in interventions.

While most middle-range theories in nursing have assessment tools that permit the measurement or identification of the central elements in the model, comparing the theory of unpleasant symptoms with the theory of planned behavior highlights a weakness of some nursing middle-range theories. In the theory of planned behavior, the relationship among the elements is relatively precise. The theory postulates specific relationships among the measurable values of each element. The theory of unpleasant symptoms, by contrast, leaves the "influences" vague. It does not specify, for instance, whether physiological, psychological, and situational factors all have the same weight in the determination of symptom dimensions. This makes it impossible for the model to predict or explain change in symptom expression over time. For example, will changing situational factors have a larger or smaller effect than physiological factors on the distress dimension of symptoms? This lack of specificity makes the theory less useful for nursing practice.

Interlevel models in nursing science

Thinking of middle-range theories as axiomatic structures, rather than as models, has obscured one of their important features. A model often postulates causal mechanisms that underlie a phenomenon. So far, our discussion has emphasized the decomposition or analysis of a phenomenon into elements. Many important scientific advances occurred when those elements were localized, that is, when they were identified with specific micro-structures. In a landmark work in the philosophy of science, William Bechtel and Robert Richardson (1993) used both historical case studies and philosophical argument to show that decomposition and localization are important heuristics for scientific discovery, and important dimensions of mechanistic explanation.[3] The strategy of decomposition treats "one activity of a whole system [as] the product of a set of subordinate functions performed in the system" (Bechtel & Richardson, 1993, p. 23). Localization identifies the subordinate functions with specific physical structures.

The gate-control theory of pain (Melzack & Wall, 1965) is an example of the decomposition and localization strategy. On this view, felt pain is the product of at least three kinds of neuronal activity: two kinds of nociceptive fibers (the Aδ and C fibers), which respond to physical damage to the body, and the non-nociceptive fibers (Aβ fibers), which do not transmit pain stimuli. The theory hypothesizes that the non-nociceptive neuronal activity can inhibit the transmission of pain signals. Cognitive states, such as emotion or attention, are identified in this model with non-nociceptive neuronal activity. Cognitive activity thus forms a "gate" that partially controls whether and to what degree damage or injury feels painful. In Bechtel and Richardson's terms, this theory treats the phenomenon of pain as the product of a system. Each part plays a different role in bringing about the overall phenomenon. The subordinate functions of the system are: detection of damage, transmission of signals to the brain, and the cognitive modification of the signals. The feeling of pain is thus decomposed into functional elements. The localization strategy identifies each functional element with some type of neuronal fiber or circuit. The gate-control theory is important because it presents a model of the mechanism that underlies the feeling of pain.

The gate-control theory explains a psychological phenomenon (the feeling of pain) by modeling the underlying neurology. It illustrates another advantage of thinking about middle-range theories as models, rather than axiomatic structures. It was difficult for proponents of the received view to account for theories that crossed levels because the micro-structures involved (genes, neurons, etc.) were "theoretical," not "observational" entities. Relationships among theories at different levels were conceived as relations among laws. By contrast, the "levels" spanned by the gate-control theory are not more and less abstract laws. They are ontological levels in the sense that they relate one kind of object or system to another. Kenneth Schaffner, who developed these ideas in the context of biomedical science, articulated this notion of a level in terms of aggregation:

---

[3] Bechtel and Richardson were building on prior work in this area, particularly Herbert Simon, for example (1969), and William Wimsatt (1972, 1986). Similar ideas have been developed and refined in more recent philosophy of science, for example (Woodward, 2003) or (Darden, 2006).

meaning .... Concepts are not like bricks, they are more like niches." (Paley, 1996, p. 577)

The most thorough development of this idea within the nursing literature has been in Beth Rodgers' work (1989, [1993] 2000, 2000). Like Paley, Rodgers treats concepts as getting their meaning from the theories of which they are part, and as a consequence, changing as theories change. Rodgers developed this idea into an "evolutionary" view of concept analysis and development. Concepts are not created ex nihilo in her view. They are drawn from existing bodies of literature, clarified, and put to use in the context of theories. As the theories are applied and developed, the concepts evolve:

> *"[C]oncept development must be an ongoing process, with no realistic end point, except that work on a particular concept may decrease as the concept loses significance. As phenomena, needs, and goals change, concepts must be continually refined and variations introduced to achieve a clearer and more useful repertoire."* (Rodgers, 2000, p. 82)

The difference between concepts as theory-formed and concepts as theory-forming, then, presents us with a choice between two very different ways of thinking about concepts and theories. There has been substantial philosophical literature on this topic.[1] The challenge for this chapter is to sort through the issues as they appear in nursing. How should nurse scholars think about the relationship between concepts and theories?

Public and personal concepts

Before we tackle the question of how concepts are related to theories, there is a prior, ontological question that needs to be discussed: What *are* concepts and theories? It is common for essays on concept development in nursing to affirm that concepts are (or are like) mental images. The following definitions are taken from widely used textbooks:

> *"A* concept *is a mental image of a phenomenon, an idea, or a construct in the mind about a thing or an action."* (Walker & Avant, [1983] 2005, p. 26)

> *"We define the term* concept *as a complex mental formulation of experience. By 'experience,' we mean perceptions of the world, including objects, other people, visual images, color, movement, sounds, behavior, interactions—the totality of what is perceived."* (Chinn & Kramer, [1983] 1999, p. 61)

---

[1] In philosophy, the thesis that the meaning of a word or concept depends on its context is often called "semantic holism" (cf. Fodor & Lepore, 1992). Since the word "holism" has already been used twice (Chapters 10 and 13) with two different meanings (caution!), we will not use that term here. We will follow the nursing literature and use "contextualism" to express the idea that concepts are theory-formed.

"*[C]oncepts are formed by the identification of characteristics common to a class of objects or phenomena and the abstraction and clustering of these characteristics, along with some means of expression (most often a word). Although concepts are individual and private in nature, the process of abstraction, clustering, and association of the concept with a word (or other means of expression) is influenced heavily by socialization and public interaction.*" (Rodgers, 2000, p. 78)

To think of a concept as a mental image or mental formulation is to think of it as a personal kind of thing. Since experiences differ among people, we would expect their complex mental formulations to differ too. As Rodgers wrote, they are "individual and private." In this sense of "concept," everyone has different concepts of pain, caring, or social support. The quotation from Rodgers suggests that these personal concepts are represented in language, and that they become similar through social interaction. On this way of thinking about concepts, they are private entities that are expressed through speech and action.

A different way to treat concepts is to take them to be public, shared entities. This is, perhaps, the sense expressed in Fawcett's definition:

"*A* concept *is a word or phrase that summarizes the essential characteristics or properties of a phenomenon.*" (Fawcett, [1985] 1999, p. 1)

Words are public. The same word (with the same meaning) may be repeated by different people. Most metatheoretical or philosophical discussion of concepts in science is concerned primarily with public, shared concepts. When a scholar analyzes the concept of a "gate" in the gate-control theory of pain, she is not reporting on her impressions. She has worked through the literature and found some attributes of the concept expressed there. Or again, to point out that a middle-range theory is inconsistent with a particular conceptual model is not to accuse any individual of inconsistency. And to articulate the difference between the concepts of "stress" in physics and physiology is not to describe the mental images of physicists and psychologists. In all of these cases, we are not concerned with private mental images or constructions. We are interested in something public and shared in the way that texts are shared. It is a bit of an overstatement, however, to *identify* a concept with a word, as the quotation from Fawcett does. The same concept may be expressed by two different words (or phrases), or it may be expressed both verbally and nonverbally. It would be better, then, to identify concepts with the meaning of a word or phrase, and this may have been Fawcett's intention.

Both the public and the private senses of "concept" are legitimate, and both have been deployed by philosophers and psychologists. Moreover, while some philosophers have tried to argue for one sense to the exclusion of the other, there are ways to make the public and private senses of "concept" consistent. The nursing literature on concepts, however, manifests a tension between the two uses. The methods of concept analysis, for example, often slip between the two senses in ways that create confusion. For example, Walker and Avant characterize concepts as mental images or constructs. However, their method requires the analyst to identify as many uses as possible, including "dictionaries, thesauruses, colleagues, and available literature" (Walker & Avant, [1983] 2005, p. 67). If a concept is the mental image of the person doing the analysis, it is hard to see how a dictionary or the literature could provide any useful information. The only way to discover what mental image I associate, say, with the concept of a "gate," would be to introspect. I would say the word to myself and note the mental images that emerge. Such a procedure would have little interest for the nursing discipline. The point of consulting published literature is to discover the public concept, for example, to find out what "gate" means in the gate-control theory of pain. A similar tension is found in Rodgers' discussion. After saying that concepts are "individual and private in nature" (Rodgers, 2000, p. 78), she goes on to articulate a method that involves systematic sampling and identification of themes within published literature. The methods of concept analysis proposed by Rodgers, Walker, and Avant, and others aim at discovering public concepts as expressed in scientific literature, even though they define "concepts" in terms of private mental imagery.

The emphasis on the personal sense of "concept" is, perhaps, a result of trying to clearly distinguish between a concept and what it represents. A mental image of an apple, for instance, is one thing, and the real apple is another. An image is also easily understood as accurate or inaccurate. The image associated with my concept of an apple might be large and red, while the apple on the table is small and green. In this case, my concept of an apple (the mental image) is not an accurate representation of the apple before me. To speak of concepts and theories as mental constructions, then, nicely highlights some of their salient features. They are constructions over which the theorist has control, they are distinct from what they represent, and they can represent it well or badly. However, concepts need not be mental images to have these properties. If we think of theories as linguistic objects, written down in textbooks and journal essays, they have the same features. As a set of propositions (roughly, the meaning of sentences) and concepts (roughly, the meaning of words), a theory is the creation of one or more theorists. It is a representation of something—a nursing situation, a physiological structure or process, the experience of a particular patient—and it can represent those things accurately or inaccurately. The advantage of thinking about scientific theories and concepts as linguistic is that they can be shared. Two theorists can contemplate, test, and disagree about the *same* theory, which would be impossible if the theory were identified with their different private mental constructions.

The aim of these arguments is not to exclude one or the other senses of "concept." Again, the public and private senses are consistent, and each communicates a part of what we mean when we talk about concepts and conceptualization. What is important, and will remain important, is to keep the two distinct. That said, public concepts will be the main focus of this chapter.

The priority of theory

The idea that concepts are prior to theory (theory-forming) has long been an aspect of empiricism. The classical empiricists (e.g., John Locke, George Berkeley, and

David Hume) took simple ideas of sensation like "round" or "blue"—what would later be called observational concepts—to be the basis for all thought and knowledge about the empirical world. All complex concepts had to be assembled from these simple building blocks. (Notice that the classical empiricists took concepts to be private, not public, entities.) Many of the arguments that concepts are contextual arose in response to the limitations of empiricism. As explained in Chapter 10, traditional empiricism is inadequate because it is impossible to explain how we can form concepts of unobservable objects. Genes and electrons are not present to the senses, so there is no way to construct or define the concept of a gene using only observable ideas. But the postulation of mechanisms that lie behind the observable phenomena is the basis for modern science. This problem led the logical positivists to treat observational and theoretical concepts differently. Observational concepts get their content from experience. The fundamental (primitive) theoretical concepts were defined implicitly by their role in laws (cf. Chapter 8). The meaning of an implicitly defined term is the difference it makes to the inferences that can be made with the theory. This makes theoretical concepts strongly contextual, for no concept entails anything all by itself. To have logical consequences, a concept must be part of a proposition, which will typically include other concepts. Moreover, the inferences that can be made from a proposition depend on the other propositions that might be available as premises. It follows directly that theoretical concepts are theory-formed. The meaning of any one (implicitly defined) concept depends on its role in the whole theory.

The logical positivists thus ended up with a hybrid view. Observational concepts were theory-forming. Their meaning was independent of any theory, and for this reason it was possible to use observation to choose among competing theories. Theoretical concepts, on the other hand, were theory-formed. This position was criticized by Kuhn, Hanson, and others, who argued that observation was theory-laden (cf. Chapter 10). After this critique, observational concepts could no longer be understood as context free. What an observational term meant was seen as depending (at least in part) on the theoretical context. Since the meaning of theoretical terms was determined by the overall context, the breakdown of the theory–observation distinction entailed that all concepts were contextual. The arguments against positivism thus reinforced the idea that all concepts are theory-formed, and most postpositivist views have adopted some form of contextualism.

Linguistic arguments for contextualism

Arguments for contextualism also emerged from philosophical reflection on nonscientific language. The French linguist, Ferdinand de Saussure, argued that the contrasts among words helped determine meaning:

> "In a given language, all the words which express neighboring ideas help define one another's meaning. Each set of synonyms like redouter ('to dread'), craindre ('to fear'), avoir peur ('to be afraid') has its particular value only because they stand in contrast with one another. If redouter ('to dread') did not exist, its content would be shared out among its competitors." (de Saussure, [1916] 1959, p. 160)

One way to understand Saussure's point is to think of each word as having a range of application. There are circumstances where one might use the word "dread," but not "fear," and vice versa: I fear rabid squirrels, but I do not *dread* them; I dread my upcoming prostate exam, but I do not *fear* it.[2] If we had but one word instead of the two, its meaning would have to cover both of these situations. And if we had three words, each would have a narrower range of meaning. Expressed paradoxically, what is said depends in part on what is not said. A generalization of this idea is that the meaning of a sentence depends not only on what it includes, but also what it excludes. "It is either raining or not raining," says nothing about the weather because it is true in every situation (Wittgenstein, [1921] 1974). Similarly, a concept applicable to everything is meaningless.

These ideas from Saussure and Wittgenstein are familiar to nurse scholars through the influence of John Wilson's little textbook, *Thinking with Concepts* (Wilson, 1963). Wilson recommended examining a number of different kinds of case to isolate the meaning of a word. Prominent among these are "model cases," "contrary cases," and "related cases." A "case" is an example of the use of a word. Model cases are examples where the word would clearly be appropriate, and contrary cases are those where it would clearly be inappropriate. For example, a model case of an "accident" might be a waiter who, slipping on some spilled butter, drops a tray of dishes. A contrary case might be the same waiter dropping the tray of dishes in a fit of pique. The fact that we would call the first event, but not the second, an accident is evidence that being unintended is one attribute of the concept of an accident. Related cases are examples where a contrasting word would apply. When, contrary to our orders, the waiter gives me the salad and you the soup, it is a "mistake" not an "accident." We might conclude from this evidence that an accident is not only an unintended action, it is one over which the agent does not have control. Wilson's method of cases is designed to provide evidence that makes explicit a word's pattern of use.[3] But words are never used in isolation. Most words are used as parts of sentences, and therefore the conditions of application also depend on the other words in the sentence. And as de Saussure argued, the unspoken contrasts available from similar words serve to circumscribe its use. In these ways, writers who, like Wilson, emphasize use in determining the meaning of words presuppose that meaning depends on context.

Scientific and colloquial contexts

Contextualism is thus supported by a wide range of considerations, within both the philosophy of language and the philosophy of science (see Fodor & Lepore,

---

[2] Of course, there will be examples where both words are appropriate. Many words contrast without being mutually exclusive (think of the contrasts and similarities between "trash" and "garbage," or "jazz" and "rock"). However, overlaps in use often tell us less about word meanings than differences.

[3] Wilson's cases are often misrepresented in the nursing literature on concept analysis. They are treated as illustrations of a completed analysis, rather than evidence for the analysis. See (Risjord, 2009) for discussion of the methods of concept analysis.

1992 for a survey and critical discussion). Dispute about contextualism in the second half of the twentieth century centered around two questions: (1) Are there any words for which meaning is independent of context? and (2) What is the scope of the relevant context? With respect to the first question, a number of philosophers of language argued that proper names and natural kind terms (terms like "gold" or "water") picked out individuals independently of the linguistic context (Putnam, 1973; Kripke, 1980). These arguments were applied to issues in the philosophy of science, and they became important parts of some postpositivist views (Boyd, 1991). While important, this debate is only tangential to our present concerns—even if some theoretical terms were anchored directly to natural kinds, other scientific concepts would remain contextual. The second question has more resonance for the issues with which we are concerned. What is the "context" that determines meaning? For example, what is the context that determines the meaning of the concept of "stress"? Is it restricted to Lazarus and Folkman's *Stress, Appraisal, and Coping* (1984)? Does it include the earlier research on stress that was synthesized in their book? Does it include subsequent theories about psychological stress? What about other disciplines? "Stress" is also used in engineering; is that part of the relevant context?

It is difficult to isolate, in a natural way, a set of usages constituting *the* relevant context. One might take this as a reason to reject contextualism entirely: there is no unique context that determines meaning, so we should not think that concepts are contextual. Such an argument would assume that words need a unique, fixed, or permanent context. There is good reason to reject such an assumption. As a glance at the dictionary will show, words are not univocal. They have multiple, overlapping senses. Sometimes these are associated with different domains, and the uses are quite distinct, even if etymologically related. (Think of the word "boil" as used in cooking and in medicine.) Ludwig Wittgenstein imagined language as an old city with streets laid during different times, regular suburbs bumping into disorderly old neighborhoods (Wittgenstein, 1953). The context relevant to the meaning of a word (concept), then, will vary with the word and the needs of the users. In some uses, the relevant context may need to be very narrowly construed. For example, when developing a nursing intervention from Lazarus and Folkman's stress and coping theory, presumably only the context of that particular theory is relevant to the meaning of "stress." When trying to understand the physiological consequences of stressful social situations, on the other hand, the context may encompass several theories. It is precisely in situations of this latter sort, where nurse scholars need to bring together multiple domains, that concept analysis and development are crucial for nursing (Risjord, 2009). To bring together, say, physiological and social conceptions of stress, the nurse scholar will have to develop a concept of stress that draws elements from both theoretical contexts. Insofar as they are successful in blending these elements, nurse scholars will be creating new concepts and new theories.

There are, then, many ways to identify the relevant context for isolating and clarifying the content of a concept for nursing science. The goals and problems of the researcher are one factor in the decision to isolate a given domain as "the" relevant context. Patterns of existing usage are another factor. In science, concepts are often explicitly defined, and the theorists who work with a given theory try to use terms in a consistent way. Explicit definitions thus create neighborhoods of usage that are orderly and well policed. But even within science, words and concepts are used without specific and globally accepted definitions (think of "culture" or "social support"). In such cases, neighborhoods of use run together without clear boundaries. Nonetheless, because academic writing is shaped by shared training and regulated by peer review, it is sometimes useful to distinguish between scientific (or theoretical) concepts and those concepts associated with a colloquial use of words. This is not a hard and fast distinction. Obviously, scientific and colloquial uses influence each other, and in some instances it may be impossible to disentangle them. The distinction is useful because many of the concepts relevant to nursing science have both scientific and colloquial uses, and they can differ in important ways. Patients will talk about the stress in their lives, for example, and this may be different from the way "stress" was defined by Lazarus and Folkman. By making the distinction between scientific and colloquial uses, we can sharpen the questions about how patient conceptualizations can be represented within nursing science.

Contextualism and realism

Realism is the idea that scientific theories represent (well or badly) an independent reality. The opposing notion, antirealism, is expressed in various ways: that there are multiple realities, that science is a social construction, or that scientific truth is relative to history. Whether we should think about science realistically has been an important debate within both the philosophy of science and nursing scholarship. Contextualism has played a role in these debates. Thomas Kuhn was committed to contextualism, and his work is often read as expressing a form of historical relativism. After a scientific revolution "scientists work in a different world" (Kuhn, [1962] 1970, p. 135). Other philosophers have agreed that concepts are contextually defined, but they have affirmed some form of realism (Sellars, 1963; Putnam, 1981). This dispute over whether contextualism entails realism or antirealism has recently surfaced in the nursing literature. In a survey of methods for concept analysis, Judith Hupcey and Janice Penrod argued for a position they called "moderate realism" (Hupcey & Penrod, 2005, p. 201). In response, Craig Duncan, Julie Duff Cloutier, and P.H. Bailey argued that contextualism requires a "relativist ontological perspective" (Duncan *et al.*, 2007, p. 297). The foregoing sections have argued in favor of contextualism. Does contextualism entail relativism as Duncan *et al.* argue?

Moderate realism

The philosophical debate about realism during the last decades of the twentieth century showed that realism and antirealism can take many forms. The first step, then, is to get clear about the terms of the debate. Hupcey and Penrod draw their notion of moderate realism from June Kikuchi (2003), and it has two distinctive commitments that are relevant here. First, "reality exists independent[ly] of the human mind" (Kikuchi, 2003, p. 12).[4] Moderate realism thus holds that theories are accurate or inaccurate (true or false) insofar as they correspond to mind-independent reality. The second commitment is to the "probable truth rather than absolute truth" of scientific theories (Hupcey & Penrod, 2005, p. 201; cf. Kikuchi, 2003, p. 12). A commitment to the "absolute truth" of scientific theories would mean that the truth or falsity of theoretical statements can be known with certainty. To say that the truth of theories is "probable" is to admit that scientific inquiry is fallible. This means that, at any given time, we judge our theories to be true but recognize that they may be overturned by future evidence. We accept them because, given the current evidence, they are "beyond reasonable doubt" (Kikuchi, 2003, p. 12).

With respect to contextualism, Hupcey and Penrod adopt a position very similar to Rodgers' evolutionary view (Rodgers, 1989, 2000). Like Rodgers, Hupcey and Penrod hold that concepts take on new meaning as theories change. Scientists decide how to construct theories, and thus determine the meaning of the concepts. But in choosing how to build their theories and develop specific concepts, scientists do not thereby determine the truth of a theory. Truth is a matter of how the theory relates to a mind-independent reality. The object of the many scientific methods is to gauge the probability of truth. Both commitments of Hupcey and Penrod's realism are consistent with the idea that conceptual meaning is determined by theoretical context. Hupcey and Penrod have thus outlined a position where contextualism is apparently consistent with (moderate) realism.

Contextualism and antirealism

In their response, Duncan *et al.* begin by pointing out the contextualism implicit in Wilson's (1963) method of concept analysis:

> "For Wilson the focus of analysis was not to create a fixed meaning for a concept, but to create a useful understanding of the shared meaning of a concept within a specific context. This understanding is similar to Paley's (1996) contention that concepts derive meaning from or within particular theoretical perspectives. For Paley, theories are the contexts that determine concept meaning and, hence, concepts shift their meaning within contexts."

They argue that Walker and Avant ([1983] 2005) changed Wilson's method, turning it into one that would "transcend context, and thereby accommodate the requirement of a product useful for empirical work" (Duncan *et al.*, 2007, p. 297). Walker and Avant, they contend, aimed to strip away the context from the concept and provide a definition that did not depend on any theory: "The outcome of [Walker and Avant's] analysis is fixed truth; concepts as measurable variables that ideally are knowable outside of context and function in a realist research world" (Duncan *et al.*,

---

[4] Kikuchi articulates this idea in contrast to nurse scholars who seem to defend some kind of idealism. These arguments arise in the discussion of qualitative research, and will be evaluated in Chapter 18.

2007, p. 297). Realism, Duncan *et al*. argue, requires "fixed truth," and this can be achieved only if the concepts are defined in ways that are not dependent on theory. Therefore, they conclude, realism is inconsistent with contextualism.

Realism and representation

The argument given by Duncan *et al*. misses its mark because it relies on a different conception of "realism" than the one that Hupcey and Penrod adopted. Kikuchi's moderate realism holds that theories are true when they correctly represent a mind-independent reality. Duncan *et al*. are invoking a form of realism that is much stronger: theories are somehow fixed and eternal. Moderate realism requires nothing more than a distinction between representations (words, concepts, propositions, or theories) and the things represented. Contextualism means that concepts get their content from a context, which may be a theory or colloquial use. Contextualism thus tells us something about representations. It says nothing about the things represented. It is a confusion, then, to insist that since the concepts can change, theories cannot be true or false of an independent reality. The theoretical context fixes the meaning of the concepts. Once the content of the concepts is fixed, they can represent something. As the theory changes, what gets represented changes, and the truth value of the theory's propositions may change. Contrary to the conclusions of Duncan *et al*., there is no conflict between contextualism and realism.

Moderate realism makes modest, but important, claims about scientific theories. Theories are fallible constructs that we put forward as probably true and subject to empirical testing. The commitment to probable truth entails that when new evidence undermines a theory, it is taken to be an inaccurate representation of a mind-independent reality (i.e., false). When the theory is modified and its concepts change, something new is thereby represented. If the new theory and concepts are supported by empirical test, they are taken to be accurate representations (i.e., true). This relationship between probable truth and the way theories are modified in response to testing suggests a stronger link between moderate realism and contextualism. If concepts are niches within theories, then the only way to change concepts is to modify the theories. We should not modify theories arbitrarily; theories are developed in response to testing. Contextualism about meaning thus entails that the only way to develop scientific concepts is to test theories. A theory can be supported (or undermined) by evidence only if its propositions are taken to be true or false, and this in turn requires that the concepts are taken to represent something real. Therefore, if nursing is committed to developing its concepts, the theory-formed character of concepts *requires* that we be moderate realists about nursing science.

Concept analysis and borrowed theory

Concept analysis is presented in the nursing literature as a crucial part of theory development (Chinn & Kramer, [1983] 1999; Walker & Avant, [1983] 2005). If we accept the conclusion that concepts are theory-formed, then there is an important caveat to such presentations. Nurse scholars should not think of their inquiry as creating concepts ex nihilo, then assembling them into theories. Concept analysis is a process by which the content of a concept is made clear and explicit. If concepts are contextual, then the concepts must already have a use. We have roughly distinguished two broad contexts of use for concepts relevant to nursing scholarship: the casual speech of nurses and their clients and the technical language of science. This means that a concept analysis must either articulate the concept in relation to the usage of a specific population of speakers or in relation to "the global state of the science (or probable truth) surrounding the concept" (Hupcey & Penrod, 2005, p. 205). Given the nursing standpoint, the *point* of surveying the state of the science must be to address problems and questions arising out of nursing practice. In many cases, the state of the science has been developed in disciplines other than nursing. One important function of concept analysis in nursing, then, is to make concepts of borrowed theories explicit so that the value of a borrowed theory can be judged.

Rodgers' evolutionary method of concept analysis was the first to emphasize a systematic sampling of the literature as the evidence for a concept analysis (Rodgers, 1989, 2000). The researcher begins by selecting a concept of interest and a realm or setting for its analysis. The researcher then tries to inductively identify a set of attributes for the concept. These attributes make it possible "to identify situations that fall under the concept, or, in other words, those that can be characterized appropriately using the concept of interest" (Rodgers, 2000, p. 91). While Rodgers' method is a salutary advance on earlier methods (and it remains superior to many later methods too), there are some difficulties. She recommends sampling across a broad range of disciplines and historical periods. However, if concepts really are contextual, then we would not expect to find substantive attributes that apply across all contexts. The concept of a fever, for example, changed when the germ theory was introduced, and it changed again as we came to understand how the body responds to infection. The concept of stress in physics and the concept of stress in psychology have little to do with one another. The contextual dependence of concepts means that the "sample" providing evidence for a conceptual claim is very unlike the "samples" of inductive methods. The context dependence of concepts means that a concept appearing in a number of theoretical or historical contexts may have different meanings in its various contexts. Hence, a sampling procedure that mixes different theoretical contexts or historical periods will yield an analysis that is thin, if not meaningless.

Rodgers' (otherwise excellent) discussion of sampling procedures in concept analysis must be tempered by attention to the different theories and domains within which a concept is used. The investigator needs to choose a body of literature that promises to be coherent and to yield an informative set of attributes. In the context of nursing theory development, this will probably be the theory or theories that seem to have something to say about the professional or theoretical problems in which she is interested. Since the meaning of a scientific term is given by its position in theory, the method of a theoretical concept analysis is to determine the concept's theoretical role. What other terms are associated with it? How is it used to define other terms of the theory? What predictions or explanations are made possible by the use of the term that would not be possible otherwise? In what causal generalizations does the concept appear? If the theory has immediate practical application, how does the use of the term make a difference to what is done?

In answering these questions, the theorist must not presuppose that there is a univocal concept that appears in all of the literature. It may be that superficial similarities hide deeper differences. Discovering conceptual ambiguities is an important kind of progress. The concept of coping, for example, has been treated differently in different theories. A good project of concept analysis would be to isolate these differences so that nurse researchers could judge which theory is the best for their purposes. (Alternatively, one might discover that the differences are not significant.) Ultimately, however, the goal of nurse researchers is to develop solutions to nursing problems. This means that the theories will have to be modified, and changing the concepts is a part of theoretical change. By making theoretical concepts explicit, the nurse scholar can rework them for her own ends.

Conclusion: philosophical foundations of multifaceted concepts

The Introduction to Part V presented a difficult philosophical problem about concepts. Some concepts have both an experiential dimension and a biological, psychological, or social side that transcends our experience. A concept like pain is associated with a kind of sensation; a pain must be felt. At the same time, there are relevant facts about neurology and cognitive processing that are not part of pain experience. How can these subjective and objective features of pain be unified into a single concept?

One response is to deny that there is a single concept at all. There are two concepts, one might say, a scientific concept of pain and a colloquial concept. In our ordinary way of thinking, everything relevant to the concept of pain must be part of pain experience. The distinctions among kinds of pain, the different things that pain might mean, and how a person copes with pain are all aspects of the colloquial concept. The scientific concept, on the other hand, identifies pain with a neurological and psychological state. It can have features that are not part of our experience. If there were qualitative and quantitative paradigms in nursing (a view to be disputed in Part VI), it would be natural to assign the experiential concept of pain to the qualitative paradigm and the scientific concept to the quantitative paradigm.

It may be true that ordinary talk about pain diverges (to some degree) from its scientific counterpart. Nonetheless, nursing cannot remain satisfied with this state of affairs. Practicing nurses encounter the patient in his or her full context, and one of the central values of nursing is to address the whole patient. When a patient is in pain, the nurse's response must encompass the patient's experience as well as the neurological and cognitive aspects of pain. The nurse does not have two responses, one objective and another subjective. The nursing action for that specific patient must manipulate the neurology and the psychology (through analgesics, massage, positioning, distraction, meditation, breathing exercises, music, etc.) in order to change that patient's experience. Nursing practice needs such multifaceted concepts, and a nursing science that develops the knowledge implicit in the nursing standpoint is obligated to provide them.

Theory development and multifaceted concepts

This chapter has cleared some of the philosophical tangles that surround concepts in science. The main point has been to argue for contextualism, and this idea goes some way toward resolving the problem of multifaceted concepts. The question of how to bring together the subjective and objective sides of a concept like pain is acute when concepts are regarded as theory-forming. Prior to developing any theory, we are set with the apparently unsolvable problem of articulating a concept that somehow links nociceptive fibers with feeling an ache. The problem seems unsolvable because we have eliminated the resources for resolving it. If we regard concepts as theory-formed, the questions change. The concept of pain already exists in many theoretical and colloquial contexts. Given contextualism, the only way to develop a concept is to develop the theory of which it is a part. The question is therefore about theory change: How do we develop our theories so that they span all of the relevant domains, integrating patient experience with neurological, biological, psychological, and social factors? Multifaceted concepts are part of multidimensional theories.

The concept of temperature provides a useful example of a concept that has changed as theories were developed. Prior to the kinetic theory of gasses, temperature was something experienced. When the kinetic theory was introduced, it may have seemed as if there were two concepts of temperature. What could the mean kinetic energy of tiny molecules have to do with the feeling of cold? Today, we move effortlessly between these domains. When the television news predicts tomorrow's temperature, we react by declaring that it will be hot. The meteorologist's prediction relied on knowledge of the mechanisms that will cause tomorrow's temperature. The viewer need not understand the theories that stand behind the meteorologist's prediction, but we trust the prediction because we trust the science. Recently, the link between felt temperature and facts about the atmosphere has been strengthened by the development of the "chill factor" and "heat index." These use facts other than the thermometer temperature (wind speed and humidity, respectively) to express how cold or hot the air will *feel*. Temperature is therefore a mature, multifaceted concept. It has a contextual home in well-established theories that have become part of our common knowledge. The experience of temperature is understood in terms that include "objective" factors like humidity.

Scholars, both inside and outside of nursing, are in the early stages of developing theories that encompass multifaceted concepts relevant to nursing practice. Pain is, perhaps, one of the most mature. Consider, for example, the following quotation from the Wikipedia entry on "Carpal Tunnel":

"The idea that carpal tunnel syndrome can be diagnosed using 'pain' is widespread, but quite controversial. Pain is a sensation and therefore is interpreted by the cortex of the brain which receives information from a sensory neuron which was first stimulated by a sensory receptor peripherally." (Wikipedia Contributors, 2009)

Wikipedia is a web-based encyclopedia which anyone can edit. It is interesting, then, that the writer(s) move so quickly from sensations to nerves: "Pain is a sensation and *therefore* interpreted by the cortex of the brain ...." Twentieth century research on the nervous system, along with behavioral and psychological studies, has brought us to the point that it is natural to think of pain in both sensory and neurological terms. This is the result of theory development to which nurse scholars have contributed. Other concepts relevant to nursing, such as stress, social support, coping, or grief, are not so well developed. While there are theories that include each of these concepts, the theories have not developed to the point that they integrate with theories from other domains or at other levels. Nor have these theories forged strong links between the relevant experience and the other, nonexperiential factors that are relevant. As these theories develop such links, the concepts embedded within them will take on the richness that nursing practice needs.

Concepts, borrowed theory, and interlevel models

Creating the concepts that will span patient experience and the biological, social, or psychological dimensions of nursing phenomena therefore requires two philosophical commitments. Contextualism entails that multifaceted concepts must be developed in the context of theories that bring together different perspectives. Philosophical space for such multidimensional theories has been opened by the chapters of Part IV. There, we used the image of a patchwork quilt to express a picture of nursing science. Chapter 12 presented an explanatory coherence view of theory structure. On this view, theories from different domains support each other when one theory answers questions that arise out of another. Chapter 13 discussed interlevel models, which answer questions about how a process works by providing the underlying mechanism. This account of theory thus permits a very different attitude toward borrowed theory than has recently been taken in nursing. Borrowed theory strengthens and deepens nursing science by integrating it into the larger web of scientific inquiry. Contextualism about concepts and the explanatory coherence view of theory structure therefore provide the foundation for precisely the kind of research that will create the multifaceted concepts required by nursing practice.

Conceptual models and the fate of grand theory

Models and theories

The ideas of "grand theory" and "conceptual model" arose in the nursing literature virtually simultaneously. Ada Jacox distinguished "grand" from "midrange" theory in her overview of theory construction (Jacox, 1974). Her usage was followed by Hardy (1978), and the phrase "grand theory" was common by the 1980s. The phrase is used by both those who regard nursing as a basic science and emphasize the importance of high-level theory and those who prioritize middle-range theory as against the abstractions of grand theory. While many nurse scholars seem to have used the phrases "grand theory" and "conceptual model" interchangeably, Joan Riehl and Sister Calista Roy took conceptual models to be distinct from any kind of theory in *Conceptual Models for Nursing Practice* (1974). Fawcett clarified the distinction between models and theories by proposing distinct criteria for their evaluation (Fawcett, 1980a, 2005a). Part III argued that high-level theory is not necessary for science. The chapters of Part IV have presented a view of theory in nursing science that does away with the levels of theory. In this chapter, we will take seriously the idea that conceptual models are distinct from theories and ask whether they have a special role in unifying or directing the discipline.

If conceptual models are distinct from theories, then we need to understand how. What is the difference between a conceptual model and a theory? The conception of theory used by Riehl and Roy was taken directly from Hempel (1965). It therefore has all the features of the received view: theories are formal systems that begin with primitive (undefined) terms and axioms, and observational hypotheses are deduced from these axioms via bridge laws (Riehl & Roy, 1974, p. 3). Riehl and Roy overlaid the received view of theories with Dickoff and James's theoretical hierarchy. Their text faithfully presented Dickoff and James' first three levels of theory. But they noticed that the fourth level—situation-producing theory—is prescriptive, and thus value-laden. On the received view, theories were expected to be value-free.

Therefore, Riehl and Roy concluded, situation-producing theory is not really "theory" at all:

"Thus, since models relate to nursing practice, which is prescriptive, the ingredients of prescriptive level theory presented here provide the elements of nursing models." (Riehl & Roy, 1974, pp. 5–6)

The elements of a conceptual model include the "values, goal of nursing action, the recipient of nursing care, and nursing intervention" (Riehl & Roy, 1974, p. 6). For Riehl and Roy, then, one difference between theories and conceptual models is that only the later specify values and goals of nursing action.

The orientation and abstraction pictures

Riehl and Roy's text vacillates between two pictures of how theories and conceptual models are related: an *orientation* picture and an *abstraction* picture. The orientation picture is expressed in passages like this:

"In nursing research the nursing model provides the basis for selecting the aspect of reality to be observed. It provides the assumptions and values about nursing, the goal of nursing action, and also the focus and means of intervention. Each of these elements, then, can be the subject of scientific research and exploration." (Riehl & Roy, 1974, p. 25)

On this understanding, nursing models are expressions of the philosophical background to nursing research. Conceptual models orient research and practice by guiding the selection of problems or making phenomena salient. They make no theoretical pronouncements. A conceptual model can guide research and practice only in the light of some values and goals. Nursing values and goals are thus crucial components of the conceptual model on the orientation picture. They set the agenda for nursing research by articulating what is important.

In their discussion, however, Riehl and Roy do not stick to the orientation picture. The also write that a "model is a schematic depiction of a theory" (1974, p. 26). On this view, conceptual models are abstractions from theories. The conceptual model is the bare skeleton of the theory, and a theory provides a more concrete specification of the concepts in the model. This picture downplays the role of values. After all, if theories are value-free, and conceptual models are abstract depictions of a theory, then conceptual models would be value-free as well.

The idea that conceptual models are abstract versions of theory was taken up and developed by Fawcett. Fawcett thought that there was a continuous progression from conceptual models through grand theory to middle-range theory (Fawcett, 1980a, 1989, p. 20, [1985] 1999, pp. 2–7, 2005b, p. 131). Starting with a conceptual model, the theorist derives grand or middle-range theories by making the concepts more specific (Fawcett, [1985] 1999, p. 6, 1989, p. 20). When the concepts are sufficiently concrete, they can be part of hypotheses used to test the theory. Fawcett argues that conceptual models are too abstract to be empirically tested (Fawcett,

[1985] 1999, p. 9, 1989, p. 2). Testing requires observable hypotheses. Hence, before any testing can occur, the concepts and propositions of the conceptual model must be made concrete and operationalized. On Fawcett's view, to make the concepts of a conceptual model concrete is to derive a middle-range theory. Therefore, before testing can occur, a middle-range theory must be deduced from the conceptual model.

The abstraction picture is tied to the received view of theory,[1] and they combine into a pervasive picture of nursing science. By treating theories as axiomatic formal systems, the received view placed enormous importance on the fundamental, theoretical definitions of the theory. On the abstraction picture, conceptual models express the fundamental concepts of a theory. These concepts determine how middle-level theories apply to phenomena. Also, as we saw in the earlier discussion of middle-range theory (Chapter 9), this picture places a premium on the consistency of the concepts of middle-range theories with the concepts of grand theory. The concepts of a middle-range theory get their meaning, in part, from the more abstract concepts. Hence, middle-range theories from different disciplines cannot be mixed, for their terms do not have the same meanings. Furthermore, on analogy with physics, the conceptual models and grand theories of nursing must form a "basic science." They provide definitions and ultimate laws that govern a substantial part of the natural and human world. We have seen throughout this work how this picture frames nursing discussions of theory and research.

The abstraction and the orientation views of conceptual models have some similarities, and this is perhaps the reason why nursing discussions often conflate them. On both understandings, conceptual models provide a framework for theorizing, and conceptual models are not (directly) testable. There are, nonetheless, two clear differences that have important consequences for nursing theory.

First, they make very different demands on the consistency of conceptual models with other theories. On the orientation picture, a single conceptual model might guide incompatible theories. For example, medicine is oriented by a conceptual model that identifies diseases with pathogens or lesions. A disease, on this view, is a bodily malfunction that is either caused by an outside agent (pathogen) or a subsystem breakdown. This framework orients clinicians and medical researchers toward certain kinds of diagnosis and treatment at the expense of others. Clearly, however, this conceptual model is consistent with contradictory theories about, say, the causes of AIDS. By orienting researchers toward particular kinds of cause, the conceptual model provides the background against which the disputes make sense. On the abstraction picture, inconsistency among theories under the same conceptual model would be impossible. Middle-range theories are derived from conceptual models, and no logically consistent set of statements could entail an inconsistent pair of theories. The orientation picture thus permits a rather loose relationship between conceptual models and theories, while the abstraction picture demands a close relationship.

---

[1] When the abstraction understanding is presented, it is often presented along with references to positivist-influenced philosophy of science. See, for example, Riehl and Roy (1974, p. 3) and Fawcett ([1985] 1999, p. 7).

A second difference is that the orientation picture emphasizes the role of values and goals. The values contained in a conceptual model make some kinds of inquiry important. They are therefore crucial to the guidance provided by the model. The abstraction picture, on the other hand, has no place for values. A model is an abstract form of theory, and empirical theories are descriptions, not evaluations.

Arguments against the abstraction picture

While the abstraction understanding of conceptual models is pervasive, it is deeply problematic. First, Leana Uys pointed out that theories in other disciplines can be "extremely abstract and very difficult to test empirically due to lack of adequate instrumentalization, without that making them non-theories" (Uys, 1987, p. 276). String theory in physics, for example, is extremely abstract and difficult to test. Nonetheless, physicists treat it as an empirical, testable theory. Similar points could be made for the theory of evolution or economic theories. Abstraction, then, is an inadequate way of discriminating between theories and nontheories.

The relationship between the abstraction understanding of conceptual models and the received view of theory signals deeper philosophical trouble. The abstraction picture holds that the meaning of high-level concepts informs the meaning of the low-level concepts, and that the concepts of a theory are independent of observational concepts. The arguments of Chapter 10 showed that this is an inadequate understanding of scientific concepts. On the contrary, theoretical concepts inform observational concepts, and as theories change, the content of concepts at all levels of theoretical generality might have to change. Moreover, by demanding that the concepts of middle-level theory be derived from the most abstract concepts, the abstraction picture makes it impossible for disciplines to communicate. Given the theory-laden character of observational concepts, ideas as simple as "temperature" or "blood" must differ as the highest level concepts differ. It is therefore impossible for scientists in one discipline to use the results from another. However, scientific progress very often depends on just this kind of cross-theory fertilization. Therefore, the same arguments that have force against the received view of theory mitigate against the abstraction understanding of conceptual models.

Harmful effects of the abstraction picture

The abstraction picture has had two pernicious effects on nursing research practices. The first was pointed out by Uys (1987) and by Suppe and Jacox (1985). Treating conceptual modes as abstract theories has led nurse scholars to try to test views that are simply not testable. Both essays criticize Martha Rogers *An Introduction to the Theoretical Basis of Nursing* (1970). Rogers tried to articulate a broad set of assumptions about human beings. She insisted that the whole is not the sum of its parts, and she denied that there are causal relationships between "man" and the environment. Rogers conceived of her own work as an abstract form of theory, and she suggested several "testable hypotheses." For example, "What feelings are evoked (by modern music) that may have relevance for mankind's evolving?" (cited in Uys, 1987, p. 279). Suppe and Jacox point out that these testable hypotheses depend on information that is not part of theory. Hence, the theory is testable only "if augmented by auxiliary claims that provide most of the testable content" (Suppe & Jacox, 1985, p. 249). Uys presses the argument even farther. The hypotheses explicitly formulate causal relationships (e.g., evocation) among parts (e.g., feelings, modern music). If the theory denies that there are causal relationships, the hypotheses are inconsistent with the very theory they are supposed to test (Uys, 1987, p. 279). These confusions have led to investigations that purport to be testing grand theories, but in fact have little or no bearing on the truth or falsity of the grand theory's propositions. The root of the problem, these authors suggest, is that Rogers is mistaken in thinking that her work is an abstract form of empirical theorizing.

A second pernicious effect of the abstraction picture of conceptual models (and grand theory) is that it leads to incoherent evaluation of nursing scholarship. When the nurse scholars of the early 1970s began to reflect on nursing theory, they identified Peplau (1952), Orlando (1961), Wiedenbach (1964), and Henderson (1966) as important contributors to nursing's conceptual models. Misled by the mid-century philosophers of science, nurse scholars have since interpreted their work as a kind of abstract theory. Texts on nursing theory routinely apply criteria for the evaluation of empirical theories to these authors.

For example, the collection edited by Julia George, *Nursing Theories: The Base for Professional Nursing Practice* ([1980] 1990), applies a standard set of evaluative criteria to more than 19 theorists. These include the requirements that theories be "generalizable," that theories be "the bases for hypotheses that can be tested," and that the theories be "validated" by empirical research (George, [1980] 1990, pp. 7–8). The contributors to this volume thus treat the work of early nurse scholars as if it was an abstract and general form of empirical theory. As a result, these theorists of the 1950s and 1960s fare poorly. Neither Henderson nor Wiedenbach, for example, generates empirical hypotheses and thus neither "theory" is empirically testable (George, [1980] 1990, pp. 74, 176). If these were genuine scientific theories, then such faults would be fundamental; they would not even merit inclusion in a survey of nursing theory. Yet, they are included because nurse scholars find them useful and important. This suggests that the problem is not with Henderson or Wiedenbach, but with the philosophical framework that has been applied to them. The writing of these early nurse scholars should not be understood as abstractions from which testable theories can be derived. If we are to see the value of this work, we must look at it in a different way.

Advantages of the orientation picture

The orientation understanding of conceptual models is not subject to the above objections. On the orientation understanding, a conceptual model provides a framework in the sense that it *guides* research and practice. For example, contemporary neuroscience is guided by the idea that every mental phenomenon has a neurological correlate. This is an assumption in the sense that it is not tested by observation, nor is it derived from some other propositions. Clearly, the theories of neuroscience are not concrete specifications of the concepts "mental phenomenon" or "neurological correlate." Rather, the background assumption informs research by making some lines of inquiry into the mental plausible (e.g., MRI studies) and others implausible (e.g., introspective phenomenology). It is therefore a conceptual model that orients the theory without being an abstract version of the theory.

Another advantage of the orientation picture is that it gives values and goals a natural role. As Riehl and Roy recognize, many conceptual models in nursing are aimed at prescribing theory. To do so they must include evaluative concepts, at least implicitly. It is quite clear that these concepts are not abstractions, nor do any other concepts make them more concrete and specific. We saw in Chapter 5 that parsimony and accuracy of prediction are common values of the sciences, but it would be absurd to think of any theory as a concrete specification of the concept of "parsimony." By guiding the researcher, not defining her terms, the orientation picture of conceptual models lets values play an appropriate role. Values, along with substantive background beliefs, help the researcher select appropriate phenomena and methods of inquiry.

The orientation picture is therefore a superior conception of conceptual models. We should not think of conceptual models as an abstract form of theory. They have a rather different character. They highlight important and valuable areas of inquiry and they express some broad, open-textured assumptions about how the phenomena of the field are to be understood. Theories are developed under the influence of conceptual models, but it is a mistake to think of the theories as specifying the concepts of the model or making them more concrete. Conceptual models are indeed not testable in the way that scientific theories are, but not because they are too abstract. To see why, however, we will need to understand more about the character of conceptual models in nursing.

Rereading the early theorists

Once we sweep away the remnants of positivism and the received view of theories, we can begin to appreciate how background assumptions and values orient scientific research. If the early nurse researchers were not creating abstract forms of empirical theory, what were they doing?

Nursing pedagogy and early theory

The first clue is that the early authors—Peplau, Orlando, Wiedenbach, and Henderson—all say that their work arose out of teaching. Orlando notes that her book arose from a 3-year project to "identify the factors which enhanced or impeded the integration of mental health features in the basic nursing curriculum" (1961, p. vii). *The Dynamic Nurse-Patient Relationship* is "the content of instruction" that arose from the project. Similarly, Wiedenbach begins *Clinical Nursing: A Helping Art* in this way:

> *"The concept and philosophy of nursing articulated in this book derive from forty years of experience in nursing. I have had the privilege of caring for countless patients both in the hospital and in their homes, and have witnessed their struggles to regain health, to fulfill their responsibilities, and to cope with triumphs, frustrations, and disasters. How to help these patients was a challenge, sometimes a baffling one. Out of the baffling ones grew my need to research for causes: why was I able to help some and not others; what specifically did I do that brought revealing responses from some and not from others; how did I use myself—my abilities to observe, to listen, to communicate, to understand—to bring about the outcome that I experienced?"*

> *"When I started teaching students of nursing, over fifteen years ago, my need to find answers to the questions raised by my experiences with patients grew more acute. How could I help students attain clarity about their roles and responsibilities in nursing without having first attained it for myself?"* (Wiedenbach, 1964, p. vii)

The projects of both Orlando and Wiedenbach, then, are at least partly oriented toward helping nursing students in some way. Henderson presents her work in more disciplinary terms. The opening passage of her book discusses the "search for an official definition of nursing," and her part in that search. However, she remarks at the outset that "Much of what I have to say about nursing practice has been presented in more detail in my last revision of Miss Bertha Harmer's text *The Principles and Practice of Nursing*, and in the ICN's booklet, *Basic Principles of Nursing Care*" (Henderson, 1966, p. v). So, while *The Nature of Nursing* was not directed toward a student audience, it recapitulated themes that she thought were important for student nurses.

Conceptualizing the nurses' role

Now, while these works were aimed at nursing students, they are not clinical textbooks. There is no instruction about how to change dressings, use a sphygmometer, insert a catheter, or perform any similar clinical task. In this sense, the works may be said to be "conceptual" or "theoretical" rather than practical or clinical. This raises the question: If these books were intended to be instructional, but they were not practical, what were they supposed to teach the students? Each of them aims primarily to "spell out the role of the professional nurse" (Orlando, 1961, p. 9; cf. Wiedenbach, 1964, p. 2; Henderson, 1966, p. v). Henderson does so in the most general way. She expresses "the nature of nursing" in these terms:

> *"The unique function of the nurse is to assist the individual, sick or well, in the performance of those activities contributing to health or its recovery (or to peaceful death) that he would perform unaided if he had the necessary strength, will, or knowledge. And to do this in such a way as to help him gain independence as rapidly as possible."* (Henderson, 1966, p. 15)

Wiedenbach and Orlando express very similar ideas about the aim, function, or goal of nursing:

> "[The purpose for clinical nursing is] To facilitate the efforts of the individual to overcome the obstacles which currently interfere with his ability to respond capably to demands made of him by his condition, environment, situation and time." (Wiedenbach, 1964, pp. 14–15)

> "The purpose of nursing is to supply the help a patient requires in order for his needs to be met." (Orlando, 1961, p. 8)

By specifying the goal of nursing, each of these theorists is trying to identify the distinctive character of nursing, and thereby show how nursing is different from other health care roles. Thinking pedagogically, as these theorists were, the rationale for this work is clear. A novice nurse needs to know the boundaries of her role. She needs to understand her place in the larger health care environment. These works tried to provide guidance.

While Henderson is concerned to discuss the origins and implications of this conception of nursing, Orlando and Wiedenbach further analyze the role and responsibilities of a nurse. In so doing, they develop a kind of map of the nurse's environment, and they position the nurse within it. Orlando focuses on the encounter between the patient and the nurse. Her analytical apparatus is designed to make aspects of the patient's behavior or the nurse's reaction salient. For example, "the nursing process" is analyzed into "(1) the behavior of the patient, (2) the reaction of the nurse, and (3) the nursing actions which are designed for the patient's benefit" (Orlando, 1961, p. 36). The behavior of the patient is further broken down into a half-dozen verbal and two nonverbal forms. Orlando's examples make it clear that the point of this analysis is to alert student nurses to elements of the situation. Presumably, once the student is attentive to these aspects of her environment, she will be more perceptive, reflective, and responsive to the patients' needs. Wiedenbach's analysis is substantially similar, as are the apparent goals of the work.

Models of nursing and models for nursing

Henderson, Orlando, and Wiedenbach were developing a particular kind of conceptual model for nursing. These models aim to say what the distinctive function, purpose, or role of a nurse ought to be. Given this function, they go on to articulate an analytical apparatus that describes and distinguishes those elements of the nursing encounter that are important for the fulfillment of this role. These include the nurse with her thoughts, feelings, and responses, the patient, the clinical or administrative environment, and so on. It is clear that this "model" or "map" is not merely a description.

The distinctive character of this kind of nursing scholarship is nicely captured by Clifford Geertz's distinction between *models of* and *models for* (Geertz, 1973). Geertz, an anthropologist, was reflecting on the way that religious systems orient their participants. A model *of*, say, a social structure is the kind of description that an anthropologist or sociologist might create. It divides the system into parts (institutions, roles, offices, etc.), and specifies the way in which the parts are related. As a description, it might be accurate or inaccurate. A model *for* something is a guide to action. For example, those of us who commute from home to work have a model for the best way to do so. The model does involve representations of distances and how different places are linked by roads, but it is more than a map. Crucially, the model incorporates goals and values. Safety, speed, reliability, ease, scenic beauty, and so on are traded off as one thinks about how to get home. Both the representational and the evaluative dimensions of the model come into play when a change is required, as when an accident blocks the main road, and an alternative route is necessary.

When we peel away the layers of misinterpretation that have been painted over the prominent nurse scholars of the 1950s and 1960s, it is quite apparent that they were not aiming to create general, empirically testable theories. They were not writing a sociology or anthropology of modern nursing, forms of inquiry that would create models *of* nursing in Geertz's sense. Rather, they took themselves to be capturing an ideal, a model *for* nursing that said how it *ought* to function and what is *important* for *good* nurses to do. They were guides for both practice and research. The particular concepts used to divide up and organize the nurse's environment alert the practitioner to particular domains, and the values make some problems important and others less so. For example, all three of the models we have been discussing make patient autonomy central. This means that finding ways to help the patient fulfill his or her own needs is an important dimension of problem-solving for nurses. The values and the analytical framework guide nursing research too. Diagnosing or treating disease is not part of the nursing function, according to these models, and therefore research that aims to develop diagnosis or treatment would not be important for nursing. By contrast, identifying interventions that help the patient meet his or her own health needs would be an important area of research.

There is a deep relationship between these kinds of conceptual models and the nursing standpoint. The distinctive character of nursing knowledge is that it articulates a perspective on patient health that is available to nurses. This takes commitment to the values of nursing. Conceptual models for nursing like those of the 1950s and 1960s try to articulate the values and goals of nursing, and they gave an analysis of the nursing role. Chinn and Kramer ([1983] 1999, pp. 36–37) pointed out that by emphasizing nursing processes, they supported the movement away from rule-driven nursing and toward a more autonomous role. In this way, conceptual models contribute to the political goals implicit in the nursing standpoint. A conceptual model, therefore, can play a crucial role by making some aspects of professional practice explicit. It thereby highlights areas of potential knowledge development for the discipline as well as the value of nursing action.

Conceptual models as nursing philosophy

Theories are tested by looking at their observational consequences. A conceptual model contains descriptive elements, and these may be tested in the same way as any other factual claim. But the orienting function of conceptual models requires that they be more than descriptions. They answer the question "What is nursing?" Insofar as they are normative and definitional, they cannot be directly tested by empirical research. How, then, are they justified? What criteria would make one conceptualization of the nursing role better than another? Now, there is more than a grammatical similarity between the question "What is nursing?" and questions such as "What are numbers?" or "What is knowledge?" They are all conceptual questions, and the latter are clear examples of *philosophical* questions. Perhaps, then, we should follow Uys's (1987) suggestion that conceptual models in nursing ought to be understood, not as relatively abstract science, but as relatively concrete philosophy.

What would it mean to think of conceptual models for nursing as part of nursing philosophy? We have already seen how early conceptual models were intended to provide a broad orientation for practicing nurses, administrators, educators, and researchers. Nurse theorists, especially the first generation, articulated the goods and responsibilities of nursing practice and highlighted important elements of the nursing process. It is philosophy in much the same sense as we speak of a "philosophy of life," or the sense in which corporations, associations, and institutions state their "philosophy." These orienting frameworks invoke values and goals, as well as assumptions or conceptualizations.

In making this analogy, we must be cautious. When a friend describes her philosophy of life, we often refrain from critical engagement. Her philosophy of life need not be mine. Pluralism is an important virtue in both the academic world and everyday life. However, if a nursing philosophy is to have any value at all, it must be critically engaged. Too much nursing literature, especially the discussion of grand theory and conceptual models, lacks a critical edge.[2] Books that compare grand theories, such as George's *Nursing Theories* ([1980] 1990) or Tomey and Alligood's *Nursing Theorists and Their Work* (1998) fit each theory into an evaluative framework, but they do little or no evaluation. As Paley pointed out in his review of *Nursing Theorists and Their Work* (sixth edition), the discussion makes no attempt to critically compare theories. As a result,

> *"the student of nursing theory is drawn into a universe without critique, without questions. In this universe theories do not struggle to define themselves in relation to other theories; nor do they have to deal with the knotty problems that other authors have posed. Instead, they co-exist peacefully in a world without analysis, without interrogation, a world in which the only intellectual challenge students will face is that they might need to read some sentences more than once."* (Paley, 2006b, p. 276)

This is the antithesis of philosophy. Philosophical ideas grow and evolve because philosophers respond to criticism by changing their views. If grand theory is to mature into a nursing philosophy, it must begin to create an intellectual environment where intellectual challenges are recognized and addressed.

---

[2] Uys (1987) is a rare exception. She treats Orem, King, and Rogers as philosophies of nursing science, and she critically engages each.

Philosophical criticism of conceptual models

Philosophical claims cannot be empirically tested, at least not directly. What, then, are the grounds for philosophical criticism in nursing? Or, to ask the question from a different angle, what would make one conceptual model superior to another? Coherence is the mainstay of philosophical inquiry. As Wilfred Sellars put it: "The aim of philosophy is to understand how things in the broadest possible sense of the term hang together in the broadest possible sense of the term" (Sellars, 1963, p. 37). Coherence requires consistency, but it must demand more. Philosophical views aim to make sense of a broad range of experience. This means that a nursing philosophy must aim to make sense of nursing practice on one hand and nursing science on the other.

We have already seen how the early theorists tried to make sense of nursing practice. They delineated the proper boundaries of nursing activity, isolated the responsibilities of a professional nurse, and provided an analytic framework. They also responded to the social pressures that were shaping (and continue to shape) nursing. To develop and grow, this kind of work needs a higher level of critical scrutiny. Nurse scholars need to ask: Are some proper responsibilities of modern nurses excluded from these accounts? If so, then the conceptual models need to be changed so as to account for these responsibilities. Or again: What are the consequences of thinking about a client's "needs" as opposed to "self-care deficits"? Insofar as these concepts are different, they ought to have different consequences for practice. Such different consequences provide grounds for choosing among different conceptual models, or better, different nursing philosophies. Nursing practice is thus one touchstone for nursing philosophy.

Empirical research in nursing is another touchstone for nursing philosophy. This chapter has argued that conceptual models are misconceived if they are understood as abstract versions of empirical theory. If conceptual models are to be understood as part of nursing philosophy, then we need to shear away the trappings of empirical theorizing. The proper relationship between nursing theories and nursing conceptual models is the same as the relationship between any empirical science and the philosophical enterprises of epistemology, metaphysics, or ethics (Uys, 1987). Nursing research makes presuppositions about the nursing process, what nursing is, how evidence confirms theory, and so on. The job of a nursing philosophy is to critically examine these presuppositions. Here, a nursing philosophy must go beyond the conceptual models of the nursing literature and look to the philosophical literature more broadly. The vast literature of philosophy provides resources with which to evaluate the presuppositions of nursing science. Nursing philosophy looks to make nursing research coherent with our other commitments about who we are, how we know, and what the world is like.

The philosophical literature relevant to nursing philosophy is not limited to epistemology and metaphysics. Philosophical reflection on values—including, but not limited to, ethics—is central to the enterprise of nursing philosophy. We have already seen how values are embedded in both nursing practice and nursing science.

Nursing philosophy must critically evaluate these. For example, respecting and enhancing the autonomy of the patient is a central value of the early conceptual models, and it is reflected in the priorities of nursing research. But what are the limits of this value? Not every possible choice of the patient should be supported, so where does the nurse's responsibility end? Here again, critical engagement is crucial to the enterprise. Nurse philosophers need to evaluate arguments that answer questions like this, and when the arguments fall short, they need to find ways of fixing them.

Conclusion: science, practice, and philosophy

To call conceptual models nursing philosophy is to embed them in a much larger project. It places the nursing conceptual models in a critical environment where argument and analysis are the basis for progress. It also puts nursing philosophy, nursing practice, and nursing science in a reciprocal relationship. Each influences and is influenced by the other two. Nurse scholars have long recognized that conceptual models (grand theory) provided a framework for nursing research. The idea of a nursing philosophy preserves and enhances this insight. Nursing philosophy articulates the fundamental values and ideas that orient nursing inquiry. If we adopt the nursing standpoint as the fundamental orientation of the discipline, nursing philosophy needs to be responsive to nursing science as well. New problems arise as research and theory progress, and nursing philosophy needs to engage these. Similarly, nurse scholars have thought that conceptual models could guide practice. This too is preserved and enhanced by thinking of conceptual models as part of a nursing philosophy. In this chapter, we have seen how the conceptual models for nursing made the nursing role explicit and analyzed the patient's needs. Once articulated, they can be subject to critical scrutiny. Are the goals and responsibilities of a given kind of nursing practice all they should be? Is the analysis useful for reflection on practice? The project of a nursing philosophy, then, is one of making all of nursing knowledge coherent. Each of the three dimensions of nursing knowledge—science, practice, and philosophy—constrains, guides, and informs the other two.

Against this background, we can begin to see the place of intellectual pluralism and tolerance. Intellectual progress in conceptual knowledge requires robust and rigorous criticism. This requires, in turn, that each party to the debate be committed to his or her position. Pluralism must not, therefore, be construed as weakening or undermining commitment to a particular point of view. Individual scholars must be dedicated to the articulation, development, and defense of their views. Pluralism is a virtue of an institution; it is the encouragement and tolerance of multiple points of view within that institution. In conceptual areas of inquiry, like philosophy, pluralism is important because the research is not tightly constrained. Even with the twin reference points of nursing practice and nursing research, there are many ways of making sense. Therefore, nursing philosophy must not rush to consensus. Having a variety of philosophical points of view enriches the critical environment. It provides a larger variety of arguments that might be critical of any given position. Since philosophical positions grow stronger as they respond to criticism, a pluralistic institutional environment makes for better philosophy. Nurse philosophers, then, must be at once fiercely critical and tolerant of alternatives. And this entails a certain kind of humility: we should expect our theories to be weighed and found wanting. Criticism is the highest expression of intellectual respect.

Part VI

Paradigm, Theory, and Method

Introduction to Part VI

The qualitative research program emerged dramatically in the 1980s. Chapter 2 briefly discussed how it arose partly as a response to the perceived limitations of nursing research of the 1960s and 1970s. The ensuing debate over qualitative research made questions of methodology prominent. By the early 1990s, it became generally accepted that qualitative and quantitative research constituted two "paradigms" of nursing research. Nursing knowledge has thus been divided along methodological lines. Some nurse scholars see this division as fundamental and, in important ways, unbridgeable. Others have tried a more conciliatory approach, arguing that different methods are consistent, or even complementary. The issue has important practical consequences for nursing research.

The object of the chapters in this part will be to disentangle the issues that underlie the so-called "paradigm wars" in nursing. There are two focal issues. First, there is the idea of a paradigm itself. Taken from Kuhn's *Structure of Scientific Revolutions* ([1962] 1970), the idea that science requires paradigms has become almost axiomatic in nursing. Kuhn's conception of a paradigm tightly integrates theory, method, and value. It has supported the idea that qualitative research was entirely distinct from quantitative research. Chapter 16 will explore the history of qualitative research in nursing and provide some background for the notion that there are qualitative and quantitative paradigms. Chapter 17 will then unpack the idea of a paradigm, and ultimately argue that nursing knowledge should not be bifurcated into qualitative and quantitative varieties. Indeed, the whole idea of a paradigm is best eliminated from nursing discourse.

Even if qualitative and quantitative methods are not part of different paradigms, there remain differences between them that are important for research practice. For example, whether different methods can be combined in a single study depends on how qualitative and quantitative methodologies are understood. Chapter 18 will critically examine the ways in which the methods have been distinguished. With a clear view of the differences, we will be in a position to properly understand the relationship between qualitative and quantitative methods and the research questions they address.

Terminological preliminaries

Before continuing, two terminological points are in order. First, we will strictly adhere to the common distinction between "method" and "methodology." A method is something done in the course of research to gather information. Participant observation, unstructured interviews, and focus groups are methods; so is the use of the Beck Depression Inventory to identify depression, or the use of a sphygmometer to measure blood pressure. Methods are thus part of research practice. Methodology is an account of method. A methodology articulates how and why the method works, its strengths and limitations, and its possible sources of bias or confound. When choosing a method, a researcher must determine whether a particular approach will produce reliable and relevant information in the circumstances. This is a methodological question. There are broader questions of methodology as well: what using a method presupposes about the object of study, whether using a particular method is consistent with a given theoretical stance, what values are implicit in a method, and so on.

Second, the words "qualitative" and "quantitative" are troublesome. It is not always clear how a given research technique fits into the two categories. We will tolerate the vagueness, for the ultimate conclusion of Chapter 16 will be that it is harmless. A more acute problem is that the terms "qualitative" and "quantitative" are ambiguous with respect to the method–methodology distinction. This ambiguity has caused some miscommunication in the literature. For example, proponents of multimethod research have touted the use of both qualitative and quantitative *methods*, for example, both unstructured interviews and the Beck Depression Inventory. In response, opponents of the multimethod research have pointed to the inconsistency of quantitative and qualitative *methodologies*. The ambiguity between the qualitative–quantitative distinction as a distinction in method or methodology is not one that can be resolved easily by terminological fiat. It must suffice to note that the main concern herein is with methodology, not method. Our questions are these: Are there two fundamentally different methodologies in nursing? Or is there a unified methodological framework within which the various methods of nursing research can all be appropriately understood?

The rise of qualitative research

With some notable exceptions, there was virtually no discussion of qualitative research in the nursing literature before 1980. By the mid-1980s, nursing was abuzz with discussions of qualitative methods and methodology. Why did the popularity of qualitative research grow so quickly in the 1980s?

Both the methods of qualitative research and their philosophical background were products of the early twentieth century. By the time nursing research was established in the 1950s, both anthropology and sociology had strong research programs based on interviews and participant observation.[1] These methods were not ignored by nurses. Throughout the 1960s and 1970s, nurse researchers used interviewing as a method, and there was some interest in participant observation and other methods drawn from anthropology and sociology (Quint, 1962, 1967; Glaser & Strauss, 1966; Leininger, 1969; Osborne, 1969; Ragucci, 1972). There was, however, little discussion of the methodology that supported these methods, and there was no attempt to segregate qualitative and quantitative methodologies.[2] During the 1980s, by contrast, there were at least 20 essays published on qualitative methodology in the major nursing journals and a half-dozen books explaining how the methods could be used.

The reason for the dramatic change was twofold. Developments of the 1970s within nursing and the philosophy of science opened an intellectual space for qualitative methodology to occupy. Once available, the qualitative methodology had several features that made it attractive to nurse scholars. As a result, qualitative research became a major part of nursing scholarship.

---

[1] For a discussion of the twentieth-century history of these disciplines with an emphasis on the philosophical issues to be discussed here, see Risjord (2007).

[2] The phrase "qualitative research" was used in the 1960s (Glaser & Strauss, 1966; Quint, 1967), but the term did not catch on until much later.

Making space for qualitative methodology: Carper, Benner, and Watson

Carper's articulation of the "aesthetic" pattern of knowing (1978) was one development within nursing that opened a space for qualitative methodology. The aesthetic pattern captured the art of nursing. It is a nurse's ability to respond to the patient in the fullness of his or her situation. Carper argued that this form of knowledge had a unique character, and it could not be expressed in the empiric pattern. Her description of the differences between the aesthetic and the empirical patterns mirrored philosophical discussions of the differences between the social sciences and the natural sciences. According to the logical positivist conception, science aims to produce theories. As we have seen in Chapter 8, their understanding of theory was modeled on the natural sciences, especially those with a prominent mathematical component. Theories were supposed to be a hierarchically organized structure of laws, and proper scientific theories were verified by testing predictions. A robust philosophical tradition, reaching back into the nineteenth century, argued that the social sciences must be different from the natural sciences. According to these critics, the study of humans must be concerned with meaning, intentional action, or human value, and it did not fit into the framework of positivist theories. The kind of knowledge developed in history or ethnography, for example, was particular, not general. Understanding what an event meant to an historical agent does not require finding universal laws. Some philosophers and social scientists argued further that understanding the social world depended on a kind of empathy (or, more properly, *verstehen*). Finally, these philosophers developed the relationship between understanding in the human sciences and understanding of art in a way that made both "instances of knowledge aesthetic".[3]

When Carper presented the aesthetic pattern of knowing, she differentiated it from the empiric pattern in several ways (Carper, 1978, p. 16). The aesthetic pattern (1) is particular rather than general, (2) is subjective rather than objective, (3) resists description in language, and (4) involves empathy with the other. All of these elements had already been used in philosophy to distinguish the social from the natural sciences. Carper's aesthetic pattern thus opened the possibility that nursing knowledge might include forms that are different from the natural sciences. However, Carper's essay did not discuss the relationship between the aesthetic pattern of knowledge and qualitative methods. That relationship was strongly forged by Benner's *From Novice to Expert* (Benner, 1984). Benner argued that the knowledge embedded in nursing practice could be elicited by qualitative methods. She also contended that representing this practical knowledge was an important contribution to nursing theory. Carper's aesthetic pattern thus opened the epistemological

---

[3] For examples of the arguments mentioned here, the reader might consult the essays collected in Dallmayr and McCarthy, *Understanding and Social Inquiry* (1977). For a discussion of how knowledge of the human world is analogous to knowledge of art, see Makkreel (1992) who traces this tradition back through Dilthey to Kant. For a discussion of these issues in a postpositivist light, see Risjord (2000).

space for qualitative methods in nursing, and Benner established their usefulness and importance.

Another development that opened nursing to qualitative methodologies came from philosophy. Parts II and III canvassed many of the reasons why many of the main tenets of the received view were rejected or modified by philosophers of science. Watson was among the first in nursing to recognize the consequences of the critique of the received view for nursing. In "Nursing's scientific quest" (1981), she bemoaned the failure of nursing science. Not only had adherence to a natural scientific model of research yielded few results, it had also caused nursing to lose sight of its leaders'

> *"call for research aimed fundamentally at the solution of human health problems. Such leaders as Nightingale, Henderson, Krueter, and Hall were advocates of an integrated approach to scientific study that would capitalize on nursing's richness and complexity, not separate practice from research, the art from science, the 'doing' of nursing from the 'knowing,' the psychological from the physical, and theory from clinical care."*
> (Watson, 1981, p. 413)

What nursing needed was exactly the kind of science that seemed to be emerging from the critique of the received view, a science that rejected the positivist model of objectivity, personal detachment, and value-freedom. Watson's view was developed by other nurse scholars who argued that a postpositivist philosophy of science was a good fit for nursing (Tinkle & Beaton, 1983; Silva & Rothbart, 1984; Moccia, 1988; Kim, 1989).

To many nurse researchers in the late 1970s and early 1980s, qualitative research seemed to be exactly the new form of science for which Watson was calling. One of the earliest and most important inspirations for methodological reflection on qualitative methods was phenomenology (Bogdan & Taylor, 1975; Paterson & Zderad, 1976). Nursing discussions of this early twentieth-century school centered on the work of Edmund Husserl, Martin Heidegger, Jean-Paul Sartre, and Maurice Merleau-Ponty. They emphasized both the subjective character of experience and the importance of appreciating subjective experience when understanding other people. Qualitative research was thus said to be subjective, rather than objective, value-laden rather than value-free, engaged rather than detached, and so on. The nice fit between qualitative methodology and nursing practice promised a form of nursing theory that would be more congruent with the goals and practices of nursing than the previously dominant forms of research (Leininger, 1985; Duffy, 1986, 1987b; Moccia, 1988).

The triangulation problem

The earliest nursing proponents of qualitative research regarded qualitative and quantitative research as consistent and complementary. They argued that there were clear advantages to qualitative methods. Interviews and participant observation exposed layers of meaning and significance that were invisible to survey or psychometric instruments, thus capturing the richness of nursing phenomena (Patton, [1980] 1990; Klenow, 1981; Swanson & Chenitz, 1982). Qualitative methods were also useful for preliminary research. Survey or psychometric instruments required the researcher to have already conceptualized the domain. If hypotheses were to be formed and tested, the researcher must already have a theory. Qualitative methods allowed the researcher to learn about a new field and form tentative theoretical constructs (Klenow, 1981). Both of these ideas were reiterated by later writers (Duffy, 1986, 1987b; Sohier, 1988; Morse, 1991) and became part of the common wisdom about qualitative research. Notice that neither of these rationales for using qualitative methods conflicted with the use of quantitative methods. Some of the earliest writers about qualitative research thus argued for the joint use of qualitative and quantitative methods, what became known as "triangulation."

Triangulation and confirmation

An early and influential essay on triangulation in the nursing journals was by Laura and William Goodwin (Goodwin & Goodwin, 1984). They argued that using qualitative and quantitative methods together in a single study had some advantages. Their combination could make the research more complete. More importantly, they argued that the joint use of different kinds of methods would strengthen a study. Since different methods would have different weaknesses, similar results would serve to confirm that the findings were not the result of error or bias. The idea that the triangulation of quantitative and qualitative methods could help confirm the results of a single study was accepted and developed by a number of writers in the 1980s (Mitchell, 1986; Duffy, 1987b; Knafl et al., 1988; Sohier, 1988).

Adding confirmation to the list of triangulation's virtues was a philosophically significant and contentious move. By the time that Goodwin and Goodwin were writing, Thomas Kuhn's concept of a paradigm (Kuhn, [1962] 1970) had already been used to distinguish qualitative methodology from quantitative methodology. Within a paradigm, methods were tightly bound to the theories they tested. Moreover, according to Kuhn, paradigms were incommensurable; they could not be compared. To contend that different methods could support a single study, then, Goodwin and Goodwin had to argue that qualitative and quantitative methods were consistent. They did so, concluding that:

> "Trying rigidly to link paradigm with method will inevitably lead to research that is conducted inappropriately and which, therefore, will produce findings that lack credibility." (Goodwin & Goodwin, 1984, pp. 378–379)

This point was vigorously debated within the nursing journals for the next decade.

Objections to triangulation

The proposal that qualitative and quantitative methods might be blended in a single study provoked a sharp reaction. Bethel Powers argued that Goodwin and Goodwin had ignored the way in which choices of method depended on the underlying purposes of the study. Since a paradigm's fundamental assumptions about the world determine what questions may (and may not) be asked, methodological choices only make sense in the context of a paradigm (Powers, 1987, p. 123). She also criticized their assumption that "science is a single-paradigm multiple-method type of enterprise" (Powers, 1987, p. 124) and argued that Goodwin and Goodwin had implicitly adopted the positivist paradigm. Had they recognized the distinctive philosophical commitments of the phenomenological paradigm, they would not have been able to draw their conclusions. Powers' arguments were echoed by Phillips (1988a, 1988b). He enumerated several differences between qualitative and quantitative research and treated them as logical dichotomies, for example, holistic versus particularistic, dynamic reality versus static reality, meaning versus causality. Because he treated these pairs as dichotomies, he concluded that combining qualitative and quantitative forms of research was logically incoherent:

> *"Blended research gives an array of data related to each method. Such data will not yield information that enhances the validity of the results because the data are not compatible. The results are invalid because numerical and textual data cannot be combined in a meaningful analysis."* (Phillips, 1988a, p. 4)

Phillips was thus arguing for the direct opposite of Goodwin and Goodwin's claim about paradigms and methods.

Two paradigms of nursing inquiry

The notion that good research required exclusive adherence to a paradigm was an important change in nurses' thinking about qualitative and quantitative research. Following the lead of scholars in education, sociology, and anthropology, early writers on qualitative research regarded qualitative and quantitative research as compatible. But by the late 1980s, nursing had largely abandoned the idea that the two kinds of method could be fit into a single methodology. This distinctive methodological stance was the result of the way in which qualitative methodology and arguments against logical positivism intersected with the goals of the nursing discipline and the features of nursing practice. Once qualitative research was associated with a paradigm, and the qualitative paradigm was contrasted with logical positivism, the issue took on disciplinary significance. Choice between qualitative and quantitative paradigms came to be treated as a major choice of direction for the entire discipline of nursing (Haase & Myers, 1988; Moccia, 1988; Porter, 1989).

Since the 1980s, the methodological debate has turned on the question of how these two conflicting paradigms were characterized and related. If nursing was to choose between two incompatible alternatives, it was important to articulate what the features of these paradigms might be. One way of drawing the distinction followed the dispute in the philosophy of science between the positivists and their critics. Bogdan and Taylor's *Introduction to Qualitative Methods: A Phenomenological Approach to the Social Sciences* (Bogdan & Taylor, 1975) described the qualitative–quantitative distinction in terms of phenomenological and positivist paradigms, and this language was adopted by Duffy (1986, 1987b). Nurses who were developing the methodological foundation for qualitative methods quickly gravitated to phenomenology of one sort or another (Benner, 1984; Allen & Jensen, 1990; Mitchell & Cody, 1992; Morse, 1995; Boyd, 2001; Munhall, 2001).

The distinctive features of qualitative inquiry were solidified by Yvonna Lincoln and Egan Guba in their influential book *Naturalistic Inquiry* (1985). Lincoln and Guba portrayed the rejection of positivism with lively prose laced with examples from politics and popular culture. They presented the key differences between the old and the new philosophies of science in a table that contrasted the "axioms" of the "Positivist Paradigm" and the "Naturalist Paradigm" (Lincoln & Guba, 1985, p. 37). In this table, the positivist paradigm is represented as holding that "reality is single, tangible, and fragmentable" while "realities are multiple, constructed, and holistic" in the naturalist paradigm. For the positivist, "time- and context-free generalizations (nomothetic statements) are possible," while for the naturalist "only time- and context-bound working hypotheses (idiographic statements) are possible." And science is value-free in the positivist paradigm, while it is "value-bound" in the naturalist paradigm. Lincoln and Guba's characterization of naturalistic inquiry became a canonical description of qualitative research (see Duffy, 1986, 1987a, 1987b; Phillips, 1988a; Mitchell & Pilkington, 1999; Boyd, 2001; Racher & Robinson, 2002; Giddings & Grant, 2007).

While the nursing literature fixed the features of qualitative inquiry in the 1980s, the quantitative side of the distinction remained nebulous into the early 1990s. Nurse scholars who were broadly in favor of quantitative methods also distanced themselves from positivism (Tinkle & Beaton, 1983; Silva & Rothbart, 1984; Moccia, 1988; Schumacker & Gortner, 1992). Hence, characterizing the paradigms as a contrast between positivism and phenomenology (or naturalism) eventually failed to make the distinction that nurse scholars felt necessary. In the 1990s, when the critique of positivism was assimilated into nursing metatheory, the distinction between the qualitative and qualitative paradigms became identified with the difference between phenomenology and a postpositivist philosophy of science (Clark, 1998; Mitchell & Pilkington, 1999; Munhall, 2001; Racher & Robinson, 2002; Giddings & Grant, 2007).

In a 2003 essay, Shelia Twinn wrote of a quiet truce in the debates we have just canvassed:

> "There is little doubt that the paradigm wars have been resolved in nursing. In general, there has been acceptance for several years of the need for both positivist and constructivist paradigms in addressing nursing questions." (Twinn, 2003, p. 549)

Twinn's assessment may have been a bit optimistic, since essays continue to appear that explore the question of whether quantitative and qualitative methods might be combined within a single methodological perspective (Racher & Robinson, 2002; Risjord *et al.*, 2002; Giddings & Grant, 2007). The question of whether nursing knowledge comes in two kinds is an important issue of nursing epistemology, and it is still very much alive—even if the debate is somewhat less shrill than it was in the 1980s.

Conclusion: method, theory, and paradigm

How tightly bound are theory, methodology, and method? In the above discussion of triangulation, we saw Goodwin and Goodwin contend that good methodology required a loose relationship between theory and method. Phillips argued for the opposite, contending that, on pain of meaningless results, theory and method must be tightly linked. Their dispute lies at the heart of our question: Are there two fundamentally different kinds of nursing knowledge? Nurse scholars adopted the idea that there were two paradigms of nursing knowledge because they decided that good methodology required strict adherence to a single paradigm. To address these issues, we must address the question of how theories, methods, and paradigms are related.

What is a paradigm?

The idea that paradigms are a central part of science was introduced in Thomas Kuhn's *Structure of Scientific Revolutions* ([1962] 1970). Kuhn argued that theory, method, ontology, and value were deeply integrated within a paradigm. As a result, scientific change was not the incremental accumulation of knowledge. The history of science is a series of scientific revolutions: noncumulative, radical discontinuities. Kuhn's ideas were important, but not all of them have endured the test of philosophical criticism. Our work in this chapter, then, will have three parts. First, we will review Kuhn's concept of a paradigm and explore his reasons for thinking that theory and method were closely linked. Then we will discuss the critique of Kuhn's philosophy of science, sifting the sound from the unsound ideas. Finally, we will begin to apply Kuhn's positive legacy to the problems of nursing research.

Components of a paradigm

According to Kuhn, a paradigm contains the most comprehensive commitments of a community of scientists. It is "the entire constellation of beliefs, values, techniques, and so on" shared by a group of scientists engaged in a common research program (Kuhn, [1962] 1970, p. 147). Because his concern was to explain scientific change, Kuhn's examples of paradigms tended to be closely tied to theories prominent before and after major episodes in the history of science, such as classical and relativistic mechanics or astronomy before and after Copernicus. Considered as a body of beliefs, values, and techniques, a paradigm has the following elements: (1) a theory or group of closely related theories, (2) an ontology, that is, commitments about what objects exist, (3) a set of methods or techniques, (4) a number of exemplars, striking applications, or standard problems to which the theory is applied, and (5) a value orientation, including evaluations of what kinds of problems are significant and standards for acceptable solutions. To understand Kuhn's conception of a paradigm, one must understand how these elements are related.

Theory and ontology

A theory is at the heart of a Kuhnian paradigm. While he introduced some novelties, Kuhn's conception of a theory was in many ways very much like his positivist predecessors. Like the positivists, he thought that theories could be specified in formal, logical terms, and that the various tenets of a theory had clear logical relationships to each other. The ontology names the things that are supposed to exist, according to the theory. For example, the ontology of quantum mechanics includes quarks and gluons, while the ontology of early atomic theory was restricted to electrons and protons. This example shows how closely ontology and theory are related. Theories in both the natural and social sciences explain observable phenomena by postulating the existence of hidden mechanisms. These might be tiny bits of stuff, such as electrons and DNA, or they might be more complex and ephemeral, such as the superego or the bourgeoisie. The ontology of a paradigm includes those objects the theory postulates in order to explain the phenomena of interest. Since the objects are not normally visible, they can only be described using the resources of the theory. So, for Kuhn, the theory largely determines a paradigm's ontology.

Theory and method

Theory is also closely connected to method in a Kuhnian paradigm. Each supports the other, but theory and method support each other in different ways. A method is a technique for gathering data. A method often involves tools such as microscopes, centrifuges, scales, or spectrographs, and in the social sciences it might involve survey instruments like the Beck Depression Inventory. A fundamental part of scientific training is about how to use such tools. Kuhn highlighted the importance of training and showed how it influenced what was counted as observation and testing for a scientific community. A method supports theory by providing the data that confirm or disconfirm the theory, so the choice of method determines what theories can be observationally supported.

The theory, in turn, supports the method by helping to establish that the method is reliable. If a method is to be scientifically useful, it must be trustworthy. That is, there must be good reason to believe that the method (whether it is a technique or an instrument) is providing reliable data. The only way to judge that a method is reliable is to already have some conception of the objects to be observed and some notion of how the technique or instrument will interact with those objects. For example, we think that using an oral thermometer is a method for measuring body temperature because we already believe that the temperature in the mouth is correlated with the core body temperature (unless the patient is sucking on ice cubes, fails to keep her mouth closed, etc.). Moreover, we have an explanation of how the thermometer responds to changes in temperature. In the light of this theoretical understanding, nurses were trained to use mercury (or alcohol) thermometers in a particular way: shake down the mercury, place the thermometer under the patient's tongue, and so on. Contrast the use of this method with a modern ear thermometer, or an infrared thermometer that does not touch the patient. We can make decisions about their reliability under various conditions because we understand how they work and what is being measured. A method, therefore, is judged to be scientifically valid partly because there is a theoretical understanding of how it interacts with the objects being measured. Theory and method are thus interdependent.

Values

Finally, Kuhn emphasized the role of values in paradigms. Two kinds of value are particularly relevant in this context.[1] First, scientists within a paradigm will take some kinds of phenomena or problems to be important, and they will disregard others. Before Gregor Mendel, for example, no one cared much about how a trait—like the smooth or wrinkled skin of a pea—was distributed from generation to generation. Everyone knew that offspring were more or less similar to their parents, but the proportion of the different traits was not scientifically interesting. After Mendel and Darwin, trait distributions became interesting because the theory of evolution needed a mechanism that translated survival in one generation to the traits of the next. This is a change in value orientation: a change in view about what is good to study, what is worth a scientist's time. The example further demonstrates the importance of the theory to the paradigm, since the paradigm's value orientation partly depends on the contents of theory.

The second kind of value orientation involves the standards by which good science is judged. Scientific results get published and accepted by the community only if they meet the community standards of rigor. Kuhn pointed out that these are not timeless. When a new method is developed, the scientific community has to reach some consensus on how it is to be applied. This involves theoretical judgments about how the method works. It also involves commitments to theoretical virtues such as simplicity, consistency, or fecundity. In Chapter 5, we saw Kuhn's argument that these are ineliminable aspects of theory choice. A paradigm must include a ranking of theoretical virtues.

Incommensurability

While there is more to Kuhn's philosophy of science, we have seen enough to understand why he thought scientific change had to be revolutionary. A paradigm tightly integrated theory, ontology, method, and value; each served to support the others. When a new paradigm arose, it would have its own theory, ontology, method, and value orientation. Deciding between paradigms could not be simply a matter

---

[1] Notice that these are both epistemic values, as defined in Chapter 5. A paradigm might also contain political or moral value orientations.

of choosing the one with better evidential support. After all, what is to count as evidence depended on the method used to gather it, and the choice of method depended, in turn, on the theory, ontology, and value orientation. Paradigms were thus incompatible and incomparable.

Kuhn's technical term for the fundamental gap between paradigms was "incommensurability." This means that there is no common standard for judging that one paradigm is scientifically better than another. Scientific revolutions were therefore like political revolutions. Radical change could not be justified by the laws of the old system, since the legitimacy of the old laws was in question. The old system had to be abolished and completely replaced. Similarly, on Kuhn's view, revolutionary change in science could not follow the rules of one paradigm:

> "The choice [between paradigms] is not and cannot be determined merely by the evaluative procedures characteristic of normal science, for these depend in part on a particular paradigm, and that paradigm is at issue. When paradigms enter, as they must, into a debate about paradigm choice, their role is necessarily circular. Each group uses its own paradigm to argue in that paradigm's defense." (Kuhn, [1962] 1970, p. 94)

It is now easy to see why the concept of a paradigm was attractive to nurse scholars when characterizing the difference between qualitative and quantitative research programs. There is more at stake than just the use of interviews or survey instruments. These methods require justification, that is, a methodology, and that is going to be provided by some kind of theoretical understanding of the object of study. Questions of methodology quickly inflate to large, disciplinary issues, and we saw in Chapter 15 that this is what happened in nursing. It needs to be emphasized, however, that philosophers of science have not followed Kuhn on all of these points. Indeed, Kuhn's concept of a paradigm is infrequently used in contemporary philosophy of science. In order to evaluate the use of the concept of a paradigm in nursing methodology, then, we need to grasp the reasons why it was rejected.

Pulling paradigms apart

The main source of dissatisfaction with Kuhn's concept of a paradigm is that it was too rigid and static. This rigidity was manifested in several ways, and a closer look at the actual workings of science showed Kuhn's picture to be inaccurate. First, Kuhn overemphasized the role of theory in determining method, ontology, and value (Lauden, 1977). During most periods of the history of science, scientific research on a given topic is marked by a variety of divergent interpretations, models, and theories. Moreover, these theories are much more dynamic than Kuhn recognized. Scientists adjust their theories and models in response to new evidence, and these changes occur as a matter of course, not only as part of major revolutions.

Second, there is an important sense in which the practice of research in science outruns theory (Hacking, 1983). Scientists may investigate a phenomenon with a single set of methods and techniques while several theories about it are debated. For example, the idea that some diseases might be caused by vitamin deficiencies was an important theoretical development in medicine. While there were debates about how to explain the symptoms, the methods and research techniques for identifying diseases and their causes did not change significantly during this period. Moreover, the changes in method that did occur were not aligned with different theories about pellagra or rickets.

Theory and method (reprise)

The upshot of these responses to Kuhn is *not* that methods are entirely independent of theory. One Kuhnian argument presented above is sound: methods are judged reliable in the light of an understanding of what the object of study is like and how the method interacts with that object. The mistake would be to suppose that there is a one-to-one correspondence of theory to method. Methods, as has already been remarked, are a part of scientific practice, and practices are open to various interpretations. An important function of methodology is to reflect on why, and under what conditions, a method might provide useful and trustworthy information. In these methodological reflections, there is no restriction on the theories that might be deployed. Any theory that tells us something about the object of study can potentially be important. In nursing, the object of study is often a *subject*. People are complicated beings; they are at once biological, psychological, and social. To rule out in advance any source of information about humans when reflecting on a method in nursing would be to ignore something potentially relevant to understanding the method and its limitations. Hence, especially in the nursing context, it would be a grave mistake to link theory and method so tightly as to exclude any theory from methodological reflection. On this point, we must agree with Goodwin and Goodwin: "Trying rigidly to link paradigm with method will inevitably lead to research that is conducted inappropriately" (Goodwin & Goodwin, 1984, pp. 378–379).

Theory and ontology (reprise)

Similar arguments have been made about the relation between theory and ontology. Kuhn overemphasized the way in which theory determined ontology. He did so because he understood theories in the same way as the logical positivists. Theories were axiomatic systems that implicitly defined their primitive terms (cf. Chapter 8). The ontology of a theory was just the set of objects to which these theoretical terms referred. As philosophers inspired by Kuhn began to look more closely at scientific practice, however, they found that the received view was not accurate. Scientists sometimes agree about the existence of a kind of object, yet disagree in fundamental ways about how it is to be theorized (Hacking, 1983). For example, in the early twentieth century there was a debate about the structure of the atom. Parties to this debate agreed that atoms existed, but they disagreed on how these fundamental bits of matter were to be described. It is a mistake, then, to think that commitment to a certain kind of entity (whether that is an electron or a patient) requires commitment to a specific theory. On the contrary, common ontological commitment makes theoretical disagreement meaningful.

Once we recognize that theories, ontology, and methods are in constant flux, there is no longer any reason to think that the theories, ontology, methods, and values must change all at once. A new method might produce data that motivate a small change in the existing theory. This theoretical development, in turn, might make a new phenomenon interesting, which spurs the development of new methods for its investigation. In each case, there is reason to change one commitment on the basis of the others (Lauden, 1984). Over time, all of the components of a paradigm might change, but there is no revolutionary moment when all change together. Therefore, while Kuhn pointed out some important ways in which theory, ontology, method, and value were related, philosophers of science have come to the consensus that he linked them too tightly. They are not so tightly linked as to produce incommensurable paradigms.

Against paradigms

Kuhn's conception of a paradigm was an important development within the philosophy of science. Like all philosophical views, continued investigation shows that they are not as watertight as the originating philosopher supposed. The arguments we have just surveyed are among those that have deconstructed Kuhnian paradigms. Contrary to Kuhn's view, paradigms are neither characteristic of nor necessary for good science. While nurse scholars continue to appeal to the idea and find it useful, there are several reasons why dividing nursing research into paradigms is a bad idea.

First, there is a mismatch between the idea of a paradigm and the philosophical commitments of nursing researchers. We have seen that, for Kuhn, a paradigm is closely related to a specific theory. Because theories were supposed to inform ontological, methodological, and evaluative commitments, the theory was the backbone of the paradigm. The problem with thinking of nursing as having both qualitative and quantitative paradigms is that neither form of research is associated with a specific theory. Any theory that makes causal hypotheses or is testable by measurements is supposed to be part of the quantitative paradigm. There are dozens of such theories, drawn from many disciplines, and they do not form any unified whole. There is no quantitative paradigm because there is no single quantitative theory with ontological commitments, or implications for methodology. The qualitative paradigm, on the other hand, is associated with phenomenology. Here, the problem is not that there are too many theories; there are none at all. Phenomenology is not a theory in Kuhn's sense. It is a broad and varied school of philosophical thought.[2] Its contribution to nursing science is best understood as a body of methodological ideas that support the use of qualitative methods. Therefore, neither qualitative nor quantitative research in nursing is properly understood as a paradigm.

---

[2] John Paley's essays (1997, 1998) contain an excellent critique of the way in which qualitative researchers have misappropriated the thought of Husserl and Heidegger.

Since neither qualitative nor quantitative research programs constitute Kuhnian paradigms, the consequences associated with paradigms do not follow. The most important consequence is the presumed inconsistency of qualitative and quantitative research. As Karen Schumacker and Susan Gortner put the point:

> *"One of the most egregious assumptions about traditional science is that it constitutes a paradigm that disallows the use of qualitative data".* (Schumacker & Gortner, 1992, p. 5)

Schumacker and Gortner point out that nothing in the practice or theory of traditional science excludes the use of unstructured interviews, participant observation, or other qualitative methodologies. From the qualitative side, Paley argued that Heidegger's phenomenology does not preclude the use of measurement when studying human matters (Paley, 1998). Thinking of qualitative and quantitative research methods as paradigms, then, exaggerates the differences between them and imputes incompatibilities where there are none.

The final reason to reject the idea that there are qualitative and quantitative paradigms is that it limits criticism and productive dialog within nursing. Paradigms, as we have seen, are supposed to be incommensurable. This means that it is impossible to criticize one paradigm from the perspective of another. Now, there are differences between the criticism appropriate to qualitative methods and that appropriate to quantitative methods, that is, interviews cannot be evaluated in terms of statistical tests. But, thinking of these methods (or their associated methodologies) as paradigms once again exaggerates and distorts the difference between them. As Thorne *et al.* put the matter:

> *"Paradoxically, paradigm thinking depicts those who adhere to traditional paradigms as inherently incapable of apprehending the nature of the new paradigm; only those who have aligned with the paradigm shift are therefore credited with being able to criticize it."* (Thorne *et al.*, 1999, p. 129)

Limiting criticism to those who already agree is a fundamentally conservative approach to inquiry in the sense that it prevents researchers from noticing the limitations of their research (Solomon, 2008). Treating qualitative and quantitative research as mutually exclusive paradigms therefore hobbles intellectual inquiry in nursing.

Conclusion: nursing science without paradigms

These arguments go to show that Kuhn's concept of a paradigm is not a good fit for the nursing discipline. And while we have focused on the qualitative–quantitative distinction, these same arguments apply to the division between the "simultaneity" and "totality" paradigms (Cody, 1995). When nurses choose a method, they are not thereby committed to a particular theory, ontology, methodology, or value orientation. Similarly, when they develop a theory, there are a number of ontological, methodological, and evaluative commitments that might be brought to bear. And a commitment to patient autonomy does not preclude understanding the biological systems that impinge on a patient's choices.

Since nursing research must investigate phenomena that are complex and multidimensional, it would be a profound mistake to insist that nurse scholars narrow their view to one combination of theory, method, ontology, and value. As Sally Thorne and her colleagues have documented, insistence that nursing research be aligned with one paradigm or another has created artificial divisions among nurse researchers (Thorne *et al.*, 1999). The rhetoric of paradigms serves to isolate researchers, insulating them from both productive collaboration and constructive criticism. On the contrary, problems such as pain management or patient education are most effectively approached with a plurality of methods, methodologies, theories, and value orientations. Arguably, it is only through a discipline that is open to the integration of multiple approaches can effective nursing practice be promoted. Therefore, to speak of paradigms within nursing is empty at best and harmful at worst. It is a piece of philosophical jargon that should be dropped from our discourse.

Methodological separatism and reconciliation

18

The foregoing reflections on paradigms are important for nursing, but they do not resolve the question of whether there are two kinds of nursing knowledge. Nurse scholars have pointed to many specific ways in which qualitative research is different from quantitative research. It may be that these are so deep and pervasive that they amount to two different kinds of knowledge, even if we refrain from thinking of them as Kuhnian paradigms. Therefore, once we leave behind the spurious talk of paradigms, the question becomes one asked by Madeleine Leininger early in the debate (1985): Does qualitative research need to remain separate from other kinds of nursing research, or can the various methods be reconciled?

To address the question of separatism, we will use a two-part strategy. First, we will survey the purported differences between qualitative and quantitative research and assess whether they mark a deep epistemic difference. Several differences are commonly cited in the literature:

- Quantitative research presupposes that there is one reality to be described, while qualitative research presupposes that there are many realities.
- Quantitative research aims at impersonal, "objective" theory, while qualitative research aims at the understanding of subjectivity and experience.
- Quantitative research is deductive, while qualitative research is inductive.
- Quantitative research is reductionist and particularistic, while qualitative is antireductionist and holistic.
- Quantitative research presupposes the values of prediction and control of human beings, while qualitative research presupposes the value of human freedom.

The first part of this chapter will be primarily concerned to evaluate the way in which these differences are supposed to support the claim that qualitative and quantitative research must remain separate. The second part of the strategy will be to assess the idea that qualitative and quantitative methods can be understood within a single methodological perspective.

Reality and realities

One of the most commonly cited distinguishing features of qualitative research is the idea that "realities are multiple" (Lincoln & Guba, 1985; Duffy, 1987b; Haase & Myers, 1988; Phillips, 1988a; Ford-Gilboe *et al.*, 1995; Mitchell & Pilkington, 1999; Boyd, 2001). While the phrase is common, there are several different interpretations of what it means.

Idealism

The first appearance of the idea of multiple realities seems to be Lincoln and Guba (1985). One of their "axioms" of naturalistic inquiry was that "There are multiple constructed realities that can be studied only holistically" (1985, p. 37). They devoted a whole chapter to this idea that reality is "constructed." An extreme form of this position is known in philosophy as "idealism": the world we take to be real, the world of cats and shadows, chairs and stars, is nothing more than appearance. What we treat as objective is literally built out of subjective, mental materials. Many discussions of qualitative methodology seem to affirm a form of idealism. For example, in "Phenomenology and science," Anna Omery and Carol Mack write: "Phenomenology holds that reality consists of meanings in a person's lived experience," and then conclude "If knowledge is grounded in lived experience and experience *is* reality, then it is important to examine the nature and structure of lived experience" (Omery & Mack, 1995, p. 141, italics in original). Now, to discuss the philosophical arguments for or against idealism would take us rather far afield. It suffices here to argue that there is little within nursing practice or qualitative research to recommend such a position. Two points are relevant to that argument.

First, qualitative research does not presuppose or require a philosophical commitment to idealism. It is perfectly consistent for a researcher to use qualitative methods and to be a realist about her subjects, their experiences, and the furniture of their rooms. In an interview, the natural attitude is to suppose that the person to whom I am talking exists, and would have existed even if I had never met her. Hence, the philosophical commitment that "experience is reality" is gratuitous.

Second, the commitment seems repugnant. Idealism is an antisocial philosophy. After all, experience is, in the first instance, *my* experience. On an idealist view, other people are constructed from my experience. But when a nurse comforts a patient, she wants to comfort the person, not some figment of her imagination. Idealism thus seems to be at odds with the fundamental commitments of nursing.

Meaning and reality

It is not at all clear that nurse scholars who discuss this view of reality are really committed to idealism. In the very same passage as the above remarks, Omery and Mack say that:

> "*It is the lived experience* (Erlebnis) *that gives meaning to the world. Those objects and events that we perceive and interact with are meaningful to us.*" (Omery & Mack, 1995, p. 141)

This statement clearly implies that objects and events exist, and that we perceive and interact with them. Therefore, reality does not consist of meanings; it consists of meaningful objects and events. To say that "experience *is* reality" is mere hyperbole. For their part, Lincoln and Guba explicitly *rejected* the idealistic reading of "multiple realities" and adopted a more moderate one:

> "*No one would argue, for instance, that Bobby Knight did not exist, or that the battle of the Bulge never happened (although there are people who have argued, for instance, that the Holocaust never happened, but was merely a political construction to arouse world-wide sympathy for the Jews). Events, persons, objects are indeed tangible entities. The meanings and wholeness derived from them or ascribed to these tangible phenomena in order to make sense of them, organize them, or reorganize a belief system, however, are* constructed realities." (Lincoln & Guba, 1985, p. 84)

Lincoln and Guba are clearly denying that tangible entities and events are somehow constructed by our minds. The Holocaust occurred, no matter what people come to think about it. What is constructed is the *meaning* of these entities and events for us. Unlike idealism, the claim that there are "multiple constructed meanings" is a sensible idea that is consonant with nursing practice. The way in which people experience health, the meaning they give to nursing action, and so on, are important topics of concern for nurses.

Qualitative research is thus not committed to "multiple realities" in any robust sense of this phrase. Cats, shadows, chairs, and stars are not constructed by our minds. What is "multiple" and constructed is the significance these objects have for us. A multiplicity of meanings is presupposed by qualitative methods, and it is easy to see why. The standard qualitative methods of interview, participant observation, and grounded theory are all ways of gathering evidence about the meaning that people give to the world they experience. Moreover, we know that people have different experiences and conceptualize their experiences in various ways. Hence, the use of qualitative methods presupposes that a variety of meanings exist and that the researcher is interested in them.

Once the claim about multiple realities is understood as a claim about multiple meanings, there is no conflict between qualitative and quantitative research. Those who want to use causal theories to explain aspects of human health or behavior can (and should) agree that there is a difference between a person's health and his or her *experience* of health. Both are legitimate and important topics for nursing research. Therefore, when interpreted in Lincoln and Guba's way, the idea of "multiple realities" represents a difference between qualitative and quantitative research, but it does not indicate an incompatibility.

Static and dynamic

Another way in which the "multiple realities" claim has been interpreted is in terms of static versus dynamic conceptions of reality. Quantitative researchers, we are told, think of reality as static, while qualitative researchers conceive of it as dynamic (Duffy, 1987b; Phillips, 1988a). This contention seems to have little basis in scientific practice. Indeed, the matters seem to be the other way around.

Qualitative interviewers almost always restrict their attention to a short period in the subjects' lives. It is very rare for a qualitative researcher to do a longitudinal study, or even to return to the same subjects after the initial project has finished. Qualitative research methods thus typically give a glimpse of the experience of a small number of people at a specific time in their lives. This is rather static. Contrary to the pronouncements in the methodological literature, those who use qualitative methods never try to describe the dynamism of a person's life and the way it changes over time.[1]

By contrast, many research programs that do theorize change are based on measurement. The science of mechanics seems to be a perfect example: mechanics seeks to explain why one physical system changes into another. Hence, it must assume that reality is dynamic. Yet it formulates its laws in mathematical terms and it uses measurement-based methods to test its theories. Nurse scholars who use measurement-based methods, whether surveys or biological assays, are often concerned with change in their subjects over time. Therefore, to suppose that qualitative methods presuppose a dynamic conception of reality while quantitative methods presuppose a static conception is simply a misrepresentation of scientific practice in nursing and elsewhere.

Objective and subjective

Subjectivity is another point on which qualitative and quantitative research are said to be incompatible. Quantitative research is supposed to aim at impersonal, "objective" theory, while qualitative research aims at an understanding of experience that merges subject and object. Once again, there are several dimensions to this issue.

One dimension concerns what anthropologists called the "emic" and "etic" points of view (Leininger, 1985; Duffy, 1987b, p. 356). The emic point of view was supposed to be a culture's own perspective on its way of life, social structure, or environment. The etic point of view was the outsider's view. Thus, for example, a description of a culture's values based on participant observation would be emic, while an analysis

---

[1] Ethnographers in anthropology were accused of the same problem 20 years ago; see, for example, Clifford and Marcus (1986) or Rosaldo (1989).

of nutritional intake or agricultural patterns would be etic. Similarly, some nursing research is concerned with the patients' or nurses' experiences, and other research is concerned with biological, psychological, educational, or sociological questions that do not represent the subject's point of view.

It is clear that qualitative methods will be relevant when asking questions about the patients' or nurses' concepts or experiences, and some measurement-based methodologies will be less relevant. While this is a difference, it is not an incompatibility. Neither perspective must deny the other. It seems like common sense to say that there is both an insider's and outsider's perspective on human activities. Moreover, nursing requires both perspectives. A person may not have an accurate understanding of her health. Hence, an etic approach is sometimes necessary to develop nursing interventions and to measure their effectiveness. At the same time, a person's experience of her health is important to nursing, even if that experience involves some misunderstandings. Nursing needs both etic and emic approaches to health precisely because health and the experience of health may differ.

Another dimension to the distinction between "subjective" and "objective" approaches to science has to do with the role of theory in research. Qualitative researchers, especially those who appeal to phenomenological methodologies, often say that qualitative research tries to approach the phenomenon in an open way, without preconceived, theoretical ideas (e.g., Omery, 1983; Morse & Field, 1995). Quantitative research, by contrast, uses existing categories and concepts to determine what hypotheses to test and how to test them. There is both something right and something misleading about this way of distinguishing between qualitative and quantitative research.

It is true that measurement-based methods use a set of concepts to determine what is to be measured. However, this is not always removed from the subjects' experience. Psychometric evaluations, like the Beck Depression Inventory, ask about the feelings, thoughts, and experiences of the subject. The difference between the Beck Depression Inventory and, say, phenomenological interviews about depression, is that the latter would represent thoughts, experiences, and feelings in terms naturally used by the subjects, not as standardized by a survey instrument. So, while both quantitative and qualitative methods may describe experience, qualitative research tries to create descriptions in the subjects' own terms. They thereby aim to create ways of understanding subjects that are very close to the subjects' own conceptualizations.

It is incorrect, however, to suppose that phenomenological interviews approach a subject with no preconceived notions. Any interviewer must ask a first question, and neither the subject nor the question is chosen randomly. The investigator has chosen that question for this subject because of some more-or-less specific ideas about what kind of phenomena are under study. While unstructured interviews permit the conversation to take a natural course, interviews are not just small talk. The interviewer always has purposes and goals. The difference is not that phenomenological researchers have no preconceptions, but that the preconceptions tend to be more general and programmatic.

Deduction and induction

The next commonly cited point of difference is that quantitative research is supposed to be "deductive," while qualitative research is "inductive" (Duffy, 1986; Porter, 1989; Morse, 1991). Quantitative research is supposed to be deductive because of the role of hypothesis testing. To test a theory, it is supposed, a hypothesis must be derived from the theory. Ideally, the hypothesis postulates a relationship between measurable quantities. Qualitative research, however, is supposed to begin without a prior theory. The theory arises through recognition of patterns and themes in the conversations or participant observations.

Once again, there is something right and something misleading about this way of distinguishing qualitative from quantitative research. It is true that some theories are tested by deriving measurable hypotheses. But it is misleading to suggest that this form of confirmation is required by any and all quantitative methods. To be sure, the mid-century philosophers of science took the derivation of hypotheses to be the fundamental model of theory testing (cf. Chapter 8). In the early stages of the methodology debates, where quantitative methods were understood in positivist terms, it was reasonable to draw a line between qualitative and quantitative methodologies on this basis. In the era of postpositivism, however, the distinction cannot be fairly drawn in this way. Postpositivists are open to a variety of scientific practices and do not insist that all scientific thinking be justified in the same way. Many scientific practices use measurement and yet are not "deductively" testing theory. In epidemiology, for example, correlational studies do not set out to prove or disprove any theory. They aim only to discover patterns and local generalizations. They are "inductive" in exactly the same way as qualitative research is supposed to be inductive. Therefore, it is no longer adequate to distinguish qualitative and quantitative methodologies in terms of a deduction and induction.

Reductionism and value-freedom

The final two ways of distinguishing qualitative from quantitative research identify quantitative research with reductionism and with value-freedom. At this point, these two ideas can be treated quickly and treated together. Like the deductive–inductive distinction, this was a fair contrast between quantitative and qualitative research when the dispute was between positivism and other philosophies of science. Some positivists did regard science as a reductionist enterprise, and they held that values did not influence good science. We have already seen some of the reasons why philosophers of science rejected the received view of theory. Our question, then, must be: when understood in postpositivist terms, is there any reason to think that quantitative research must be reductionist or value-free?

Reductionism has been the topic of a large and complicated debate in the philosophy of science. To canvas the details would take us too far afield. We may simply note that postpositivists have a variety of stances toward reductionism, and many who would valorize quantitative methods are antireductionist (Dupre, 1993; Kincaid & McKitrick, 2007). As for value-freedom, we saw in Chapter 5 that the question for contemporary philosophy of science is not whether values influence science, but how. Therefore, insofar as the contemporary argument over qualitative and quantitative methodologies takes place in postpositivist context, these two ways of drawing the distinction (reductionist vs. holist and value-laden vs. value-free) are not satisfactory.

The unity of nursing knowledge

In this chapter, we have surveyed five different ways in which qualitative and quantitative methodologies are supposed to be different. The question was whether these differences amount to two different forms of knowledge. The conclusion must be that they do not. The purported differences either fail to mark a distinction at all (especially when considered in postpositivist terms), or they mark a difference, but do not show that quantitative and qualitative methods have conflicting presuppositions. Therefore, the commonly cited differences between qualitative and quantitative research do not show that there are two kinds of nursing knowledge.

Reconciling qualitative and quantitative research

Thus far, we have not seen any grounds for dividing nursing knowledge into qualitative and quantitative kinds. In Chapter 16, we saw that it is inappropriate to think of qualitative and quantitative research as different paradigms. Theory and method need not be linked so tightly as to force researchers to choose between whole constellations of theory, method, value, and ontology. So far, this chapter has argued that the specific differences between qualitative and quantitative methods do not require or presuppose separatism. The presuppositions of the methods are perfectly consistent. But, if there is a unified and inclusive way to think about the methodology of nursing research, what is it?

Nurses who embark on research programs often struggle with their choice of methods. The current view in nursing is that decisions about whether to use qualitative or quantitative methods require paradigm-level choices about big issues such as ontology, theory structure, and nursing values. The arguments of the foregoing chapters have deflated these choices and made them more manageable. This has two specific practical consequences: methodological decisions are always local choices, and good methodology does not require purity of method.

Methods as bridges

Methods are the bridge between theory, on the one hand, and the people, objects, events, or processes to be studied on the other. Methods are also practical activities, and expertise in their use is a kind of know-how. Using a method is a way for the researcher to put herself into the world of the research, to be among the people she will come to understand, or to experience the objects of her study. If successful, the activities will yield information leading to a deeper understanding. Methods are not prefabricated algorithms for generating data; the researcher must build and use the bridge herself, mindful of the specific context of her inquiry.

To build a bridge between theory and the world, the researcher needs to consider both where the bridge is coming from and where it is going to. Both of these are specific to the research project. When choosing methods, the researcher needs to ask how her activities will provide information or experience relevant to the theory she wants to develop. To answer this question, the researcher needs to attend to three things: (1) existing knowledge about the people, objects, events, or processes to be studied, (2) the questions to be asked about them, understood in their theoretical or practical context, and finally (3) the characteristics of the methods themselves. To think through the matter in this way is to develop a methodology for one's research, and it is something that every researcher must do.

The objective support

One end of the methodological bridge is always anchored in the people, objects, events, and processes to be studied. It is crucial, then, for the investigator to learn as much as she can about them before beginning her research. This is true even when the questions asked and method used are very open-ended. In the "paradox of comfort" (Morse *et al.*, 1996), for example, Morse *et al.* asked their subjects to "tell their stories" and let them do so with minimal interruption. Since the subjects had experienced significant trauma or illness, they were people with dramatic stories to tell. By asking for stories and minimizing interruption, she was assuming that the subjects' accounts would take the form of narratives and that the subjects would organize these narratives in their own way.

This knowledge of the subjects is, perhaps, little more than common sense, but it is no less important for that. If these facts were not already known about the subjects, the method would make no sense. Knowledge of the subjects becomes more important as the methods become more interactive. When using a structured interview or a survey instrument, the researcher has to know that the questions will be understood in the way she intends. When measuring blood pressure, the researcher has to know how the subjects' blood pressure changes in response to daily activities. Hence, the choice of any of these methods depends heavily on the specific features of the people, objects, events, and processes to be studied. One reason why a literature review is part of every research project is that it helps the researcher understand the subject to be studied, and thus make informed methodological decisions.

The query support

The other end of the methodological bridge is anchored in the questions the researcher is asking (Goodwin & Goodwin, 1984; Duffy, 1987b). Scholars do not develop theory randomly; they do so because they have particular interests or problems to be solved. These interests will motivate the specific questions to be asked in the research. Both the interests and the questions are embedded in a larger understanding that frames the research. This might be a middle-range theory and a nursing intervention to be tested. It might be a borrowed theory and curiosity about how it applies to nursing phenomena. Or it might be the simple desire to understand more about the experience of a population of patients. In each case, the larger context serves both to focus the particular questions and to provide their significance.

Refining a question does not require making it narrower: it makes clear what sort of information would be required to answer it. For example, we might wonder whether an existing theory of health behavior correctly describes a novel population. Refining this question will be a matter of finding an aspect of that population for which the theory is a prima facie bad fit, since looking at areas where the theory seems to work will hardly provide a test. On the other hand, a researcher might assume that the theory accurately describes the health behavior of a given population, and then wonder whether an intervention based on that theory could be effective. Here, it would be wise to pick an aspect of health behavior that seems accurately described by the theory. The specific questions will concern the details of the intervention, and whether it changes the patient behavior. On the theoretical side of the methodological bridge, then, the important issue is whether a particular method will provide information that will answer the most interesting and important questions.

Method in the middle

Whether the method will provide such information, of course, depends on the details of the method itself. The fundamental problem of methodology, then, is a problem of fitting together the puzzle pieces: the question asked, the subject of inquiry, and the engagement with the subject that gathers information relevant to the question. Methods are practical activities that link the questions to be asked with the specific characteristics of the people, objects, events, or processes to be studied. The right methods are precisely those that will provide information to answer the questions. Therefore, the researcher needs to carefully consider how the method will interact with the subjects. How will her activities create the evidence? How will it change the object of study? What are the likely disruptions or confounds that will make the method useless? What are the limitations of the method? What is it *not* telling you? The methodological literature, such as the standard textbooks on qualitative methods, gives good advice about the methods, but it cannot answer these questions for the researcher. In the end, the questions and answers are her own. She has to be confident that *her* questions about *her* subject will be reliably answered by the information gained through a particular method. This is the sense in which the choice of methods is always a local problem.

Conclusion: local methodological decision-making

In our survey of the paradigm wars, we saw that both sides agreed on the importance of consistency in methodological choices. In the subsequent discussion, we have seen how this consistency cannot be a simple matter of choosing among paradigms. Consistency is indeed important, but it is a matter of linking the subjects, the theory, and the questions asked within a specific research context. In this light, it becomes clear that the demand for consistency is not and should not be a demand for methodological purity. There is no reason to suppose, in advance, that only one method will answer the research questions. Given the details of the subject matter, it could be that two or more methods will be needed. Of course, by the same token, there is no reason to suppose that two methods will always be necessary either. Like other methodological issues, the question of whether to "triangulate" with multiple methods depends entirely on the local details. Methods are many and should be used in the service of specific questions and empirical situations, not chosen in a vacuum.

A final reason to reject the idea that nursing knowledge has distinct qualitative and quantitative forms is that it distorts the methodological decisions that any investigator must make. To suppose that there are qualitative and quantitative forms of nursing knowledge is to presuppose that methodological decisions are global. In this perspective, choosing a methodology is portrayed as a decision about one's fundamental evaluative and ontological commitments. It asks the researcher to make up her mind about philosophical questions such as whether humans have free will or whether psychology can be reduced to biology. These are important questions, but they do not move the research enterprise forward. The global perspective hides the crucial methodological issues: What is the specific question of the research? What is already known about the subject matter? And, given what is already known, what techniques will most reliably gather information that is relevant to answering those questions? To divide nursing knowledge into empirical and aesthetic patterns, phenomenological and postpositivist paradigms, or to force any similar global rubric on scholarly practice is a sleight of hand. It deflects attention at the moment when the real action is to happen.

As long as the differences are not exaggerated, labeling methods as "qualitative" and "quantitative" is harmless. But it is also pointless. To know that a method yields stories or numbers is not very useful when thinking through methodological issues. There are many methods, each with its own strengths and weaknesses. The questions of methodology are not global questions. They are local questions about which methods fit the research best. Nursing knowledge does not neatly divide into two kinds, each with its own ontology, methods, theories, and values. Understood from the perspective of this work, nursing knowledge is a unified structure, a patchwork quilt of research practices.

Part VII
Conclusion

Redrawing the map

During the 1970s, the path to nursing science turned toward grand theory. Blazed by the leading metatheorists of the time, it followed the terrain of the then-dominant philosophy of science. The philosophical landscape has since changed, but the course of the philosophical debates among nurse scholars continues to follow old landmarks. Frustration about the relevance gap has arisen because of the mismatch between the directions of the old mapmakers and the new reality on the ground. At the outset of this work, we asked whether a different direction could have been taken, and if so, how nursing science might be differently conceived. The foregoing chapters have shown how the philosophy of science that supports nursing research could be different. And not only *could* different choices have been made, they *were* made. As we have unpacked the philosophical issues within nursing science, we have repeatedly encountered the work of nurse scholars who challenged the consensus. They responded to the changing philosophical landscape by cutting new trails. The result is a profusion of claims for new methodologies or paradigms. It is time to redraw the map.

Theory

Perhaps the most important shift in reference points for thinking about nursing science has concerned the idea of "theory." Discussions of theory in the nursing literature tend to depict a monolithic view of theory: a hierarchy of law-like propositions. Intellectual products that do not fit this rubric tend to be either marginalized as non-nursing theory (interlevel models) or split off into a separate paradigm (qualitative research). The foregoing chapters have tried to carefully work through the philosophical assumptions about theory. We have found no good philosophical reason why all theories must have an axiomatic logical structure. Moreover, the received view has caused—and continues to cause—much mischief in nursing scholarship.

Rather than trying to force all of the products of nursing inquiry into a single mold, we need to recognize their variety. The foregoing chapters have identified several different intellectual projects in nursing. Theoretical models, interlevel models, philosophies of nursing, intervention and outcome research, and qualitative interpretations have all been discussed. But there is no reason to suppose that these are the only alternatives. We have not had occasion to discuss assessment of nursing education or management, nor the many kinds of generalizations that may be discovered through survey research or epidemiological methods. These too are important kinds of theory within nursing science. The foregoing chapters have provided a philosophical framework within which these distinct intellectual projects contribute to nursing knowledge, without artificially assimilating them. Recognizing many different kinds of inquiry has an important consequence. It changes the questions to be asked about nursing theory. In particular, it changes the criteria by which the intellectual enterprises of nursing are evaluated.

Criteria for theory evaluation

Published criteria for theory evaluation within nursing tend to use very broad and abstract terms. For example, in a recent discussion of theory evaluation, Fawcett and Parse compared their published criteria (Fawcett, 2005b; Parse, 2005). The criteria are largely similar. Both authors list clarity, logical consistency, and simplicity. While Fawcett's criteria include testability, Parse makes a point of not asking about testability per se on the grounds that the "language used to describe [Fawcett's] criteria is slanted toward validation of theory through quantitative research methods and evidence-based practice" (Parse, 2005, p. 137). Rather, she asks whether the theory is "used as a guide for research" and whether publications have emanated from it (Parse, 2005, p. 136).

Both Fawcett's and Parse's criteria are striking for their generality and abstract character. Because the suggested criteria are so abstract, knowing that a theory satisfies them provides very little guidance. For example, it is awfully easy for a theory to be used as a guide for research. Philosophical writing and fiction have both guided research, but we do not take the research to somehow "support" the literary work. Or again, consistency and testability are important features of a theory, but they are minimal criteria. Patently inconsistent and untestable theories are rarely taken seriously in any branch of science. A nurse scholar with research question or a practitioner with practical questions needs to know more.

The distinctiveness of nursing theory has been a persistent concern in the discipline, and both Parse's and Fawcett's criteria address it. Fawcett asks whether the metaparadigm concepts and "the conceptual model from which the theory is derived" are explicit (Fawcett, 2005b, p. 132). Parse, too, looks toward the most abstract and general realms to provide unity. She asks whether the assumptions and concepts "refer to the human-universe-health process," and to what nursing paradigm the theory corresponds (Parse, 2005, p. 137). These criteria are also troublesome for reasons we have already discussed in some detail. They severely limit the range of possible nursing theories. They exclude much useful and important work as external to nursing, or even treat it as "bad science" (Phillips, 1995).

Both Fawcett and Parse demand that nursing research be derived from or refer to conceptual models. This has been one of the forces that created the relevance gap. Nurse scholars who are working on questions and problems that arise directly from nursing practice have not found such connections to be useful. As a result, reference to nursing paradigms or conceptual models is not prominent in empirical nursing studies (Silva, 1986; Donaldson, 2000). To require theoretical links as a criterion of evaluation—especially in the apparent absence of any scientific utility to such links—underscores the mismatch between the needs of nurse scientists and the prevalent philosophical views about science.

A new perspective on theory

The only difference among kinds of theory that Fawcett's and Parse's criteria recognize is the level of abstraction. When we free ourselves from the cluster of philosophical commitments that stand behind such criteria, the real differences among kinds of theory become apparent. This work has argued for a new philosophical perspective, and from it, new questions about nursing theories emerge.

The pragmatic point of scientific theory is to answer questions and resolve problems. We have used this pragmatism as the basis for a view about theory structure. Propositions of a theory are linked by questions and answers. A theoretical proposition is either the answer to a question or the subject of further questions. If we think of answers to questions (especially why-questions) as explanations, this is an explanatory coherence view of theory. The propositions of a theory hang together insofar as each either explains or is explained by another.

Because science is a systematic endeavor, theories typically answer two kinds of questions: those that arise from experience and those that arise from other theories. "Experience" is here intended as a broad notion. It encompasses everything from the carefully manipulated observations of an experiment to surveys, unstructured interviews, and fully embodied participation. These various kinds of observation give rise to questions: Why is a particular pattern found in the results? What did she mean when she said or did ...? Theory is the systematic attempt to answer questions arising from experience. The second kind of question arises from other theories. This occurs when one theory generates questions that can be answered by another. These explanations link theories of the same level. In nursing, middle-range theories are often created from the intersection of existing theories. When this happens, nursing research is strengthening the knowledge base by forging links among theories. When explanations link theories at different levels of analysis, as we saw in the earlier discussions of pain research, powerful interlevel models emerge.

All scientific theories answer questions that arise from experience and from other theories. A professional discipline like nursing must answer questions that arise from a third direction: practice. Practice is more than another domain of possible observation. Nurse scholars are not charged with merely explaining patterns of nurse behavior or client response; they must address the problems that arise in the course of nursing. These questions, those that arise from the nursing standpoint, make nursing science distinctive.

Thinking about theories in terms of questions and answers significantly shifts the evaluation of theory away from its form to what it can do. The diversity of theories emerges when we recognize that theories answer different kinds of questions. Because the questions are different, theories can do different things for nursing. If we examine the sorts of theory that we have discussed in the foregoing chapters, we can see how this changes the way in which theories are evaluated.

Evaluating theoretical models

Theoretical models decompose a phenomenon into elements or stages, and describe how the elements (stages) are related. This kind of analysis must have a purpose for nurses, so the first question about a theoretical model is whether (and to what degree) it is helpful to nurses and nursing clients. There are at least two ways in which the model might be useful. First, it might provide a kind of conceptual map of the phenomenon or process. It is useful insofar as it helps nurses know what to expect and to prepare appropriate responses. (The theory of chronic sorrow might be an example of this sort of theory.) Where the phenomenon is a causal process, the relationships expressed by the theoretical model might take the form of mechanical connections or causal pathways. These models are useful when nurses (or clients) need to manipulate the psychological, biological, or social dimensions of health. (The theory of unpleasant symptoms might be an example of this sort of model.)

Both causal and noncausal theoretical models need to be evaluated in terms of their relationship to experience and to other theories. For example, because it describes a psychological pattern, the theory of chronic sorrow ought to be related to psychological theories of emotion and cognition. These theories might help answer questions that arise from the theory (e.g., Why does chronic sorrow have these stages? Why are those sorts of events triggers?). The theory of chronic sorrow is strengthened as these questions are answered. Causal models raise different kinds of intertheoretic questions. The theory of unpleasant symptoms claims that the dimensions of symptom experience are causally affected by social, psychological, and biological factors. We would expect such causal claims to be backed up by research in related fields. The research on pain thus supports the theory of unpleasant symptoms, but since pain is only one symptom, more support of this kind is required.

Both causal and noncausal theoretical models also need to be supported directly by evidence. Theoretical models analyze the phenomenon or process into elements. Nurse scholars ought to ask: Why *this* analysis? Are other analyses possible? What evidence leads us to prefer one analysis over another? In general, a theoretical model explains some pattern discovered in experience (which might be clinical experience, interviews, survey, or experiment). The analysis into elements or stages explains why the pattern is found. The questions about the decomposition, then, ask whether the model is the *best* explanation of the evidence.

In our earlier discussion of the theory of unpleasant symptoms (Chapter 13) we noted an important limitation of the theory. While it analyzes the phenomenon of symptom experience into parts and postulates causal interactions among them, it has provided no account of the mechanisms or processes that underlie these inter-actions. Causal theoretical models, then, have a further dimension of evaluation: Can the processes and elements of the model be *localized*? Here again, support from theories in other disciplines can be helpful. The gate-control theory of pain sup-ported Johnson's model (discussed in Chapter 11) by providing a plausible under-lying mechanism. The lack of such a mechanism for the theory of unpleasant symp-toms does not eliminate it from consideration by nurses, but it does point in an important direction for future research. As the theoretical model develops into an interlevel model, we can expect the original analysis to evolve, strengthening the model and the interventions it supports.

Evaluating intervention research

Intervention research, such as the pain intervention discussed in Chapter 12 (Friesner *et al.*, 2006), needs to be evaluated in somewhat different terms. Research about nursing actions and interventions is directly responsive to the problems of practice. All of the ways in which nursing action are evaluated are therefore rele-vant here. What are the outcomes of the intervention relative to other procedures? What are the costs to the patient, to the nursing staff, to the institution? Are there issues about access to or distribution of care that are raised by the potential inter-vention? Does the intervention support patient autonomy?

Chapter 12 argued that intervention research is different from theory testing. In general, interventions are not derived directly from the theory. As a result, their fail-ure does not threaten to falsify the theory. Rather, the intervention is made plausible or suggested by a theory or theoretical model. The question of theoretical support for intervention research, then, is: How plausible is the intervention, given the the-ory? Does the theory provide a robust account of how and why the intervention would work? As these questions are answered, the researcher will have a better sense of the limitations and possibilities of the intervention.

Evaluating interpretations

Interpretations raise yet another set of evaluative questions. An interpretation is the result of an inquiry into meaning or experience. Interviews and participant ob-servation are typical ways of gathering relevant information, but as Chapter 18 ar-gued, there is often good reason to add information from other sources as well. In nursing, interpretations identify themes, ways that the subjects conceptualize their experiences, and descriptions of those experiences. In the other examples of the-ory evaluation, we have seen three relevant dimensions of evaluation: relation to experience, relation to other theories, and relation to practice. Interpretations are evaluable in all of these ways. Qualitative researchers do not like to talk in terms of evidence and observation, since these terms smack of empiricism. Nonethe-less, there is an evidential basis for interpretation: the interviews or the participant observation. The evidential evaluation of an interpretation, then, asks whether the themes or descriptions are the best way to make sense of what the subjects said and did. Are there other themes that might better account for the interview texts?

Interpretations of patient experiences need to respond to practice just as other forms of theory do, but again they do so in their own way. An interpretation should help professional nurses understand particular patient populations, the way in which the patients conceptualize their environment, and the particular challenges and barriers they face. In these and other ways, nurses ought to be able to learn from interpretations. In addition, many theoretical models have gotten their start from interpretive research, just as Quint-Benoliel did (cf. Chapter 11). So, a further criterion for the evaluation of interpretive research is whether the themes or descriptions of experience might generalize in interesting ways.

Finally, relationships between interpretations and other theories should not be overlooked. The ways in which individuals experience their environment and conceptualize those experiences are influenced by their social and cultural background. And since experience is always embodied, we would expect physiology to play a role in shaping experience too. An interpretation thus raises questions that can be answered by other theories. If social, psychological, or biological theories can help explain why a client population has distinctive experiences or creates particular meanings around an event, it strengthens the interpretation. In addition, interpretive research can help answer questions that arise from survey or intervention research. Because interviews provide richly detailed information, they have the power to identify and explain differences among subjects that are obscured by other forms of inquiry. Once we dispense with the idea that there is some kind of incompatibility between qualitative and quantitative methods (or, heaven forefend, paradigms), interpretive results can be integrated into the larger web of nursing theory.

New questions about nursing theory

The philosophical framework developed in the foregoing chapters thus changes the way in which theory is criticized and evaluated. Rather than looking at formal criteria such as consistency and testability, the approach suggested here looks for concrete and substantive evaluations in three areas: the relation of the theory to the evidence (broadly conceived), the relation of the theory to other theories (perhaps from other disciplines), and the relation of the theory to nursing practice. In this section, we have surveyed some of the forms that theory might take, and we have seen how theory evaluation along these dimensions is determined by the particular purposes and content of the theory. Similar points were made in Chapter 18 about method. Evaluation of both method and theory, if it is to be substantive, must be attentive to the specifics of the questions being asked, the kind of knowledge needed by the profession, what is already known about the subjects, and related theories from other domains.

Professional values and disciplinary knowledge

Theory was the first major landmark to shift as we have redrawn the map of nursing knowledge. Professional values are the second. The fundamental idea of this work is that the profession of nursing has a window onto human health that is not available—or not easily available—from other points of view. Chapters 6 and 7 argued that the professional role of nurses put them in this epistemic position. Professional nurses are required to work in two worlds. They must move easily within the biomedical world of the physician. At the same time, they must be attentive to the patient's experience and environment. The biomedical perspective is not mistaken, it is partial, and the nursing standpoint emerges from the effort to achieve a more complete view. However, the distinctive knowledge available to nurses can only be brought to light through research committed to political and moral values. In particular, nurse scholars need to be committed to patient autonomy and patient advocacy, as well as the value of nursing itself. These values make the phenomena of nursing important and motivate the way that questions are asked. Nursing values also inform the concepts of nursing inquiry, including concepts like health, well-being, and self-care. The nursing standpoint is thus fundamental to nursing knowledge.

The nursing standpoint opens new ways of addressing a question that has pestered nursing scholars for decades: What is nursing science? The consensus of the 1970s looked to the metaparadigm to answer this question. In the foregoing chapters, we have seen many problems that arise from this answer. It isolates nursing inquiry from other domains, and it has contributed to the theory–practice gap. Moreover, the themes and concepts of the metaparadigm do not seem to capture the distinctive character of nursing science. They are so general that many health science research programs could fit within them. Eliminating the metaparadigm leaves nursing with nothing but a patchwork quilt of theories, as Cody put it (Cody, 1999). Consider again Afaf Meleis' image of twenty-first century nursing science:

> *"As nurses and societies become comfortable with the uniqueness of what nurses can offer, knowledge for nursing will then be knowledge for health care in general. It will be knowledge developed and utilized collaboratively by members of a number of disciplines. Therefore, nursing theories will become theories for health care, developed by nurses, physicians, occupational therapists, and others. There will no longer be nursing theories. There will be theories about health care, some of which are developed by nurses."* (Meleis, 1992, p. 115)

From the perspective of those committed to the nursing metaparadigm, this is a very troubling picture of the discipline. Nursing science seems to have no unity or distinctness at all. So, in spite of the problems, nurses have not seen an alternative way of identifying nursing science.

This work has embraced the image of nursing science as a patchwork quilt. By changing the philosophical understanding of theory and method, we can find strength in the links among theories. The identity of the theories as nursing theories is constituted by their relation to practice. The idea of the nursing standpoint thus changes the questions we ask about the distinctive character of nursing theory and the unity of the nursing discipline. The focus is shifted from unique nursing content to unique nursing function. Nursing knowledge responds to the needs of professional nursing. The questions we need to ask about any piece of health research, then, are not about its relation to the nursing metaparadigm. Rather, we need to ask whether it addresses—proximately or remotely—questions and problems that arise from nursing practice. If there are common themes to nursing research, it is a consequence of the common needs and values of nursing professionals. On the view defended in this work, Meleis' description reappears as the image of a robust and vital science.

In Chapter 1, we saw that one of the reasons nurses sought to develop a research program was to help defend the profession against unwanted changes. This was part of the reason why nurse scholars thought that the discipline should "govern" the profession (Johnson, 1959a; Donaldson & Crowley, 1978). Another way in which the perspective presented in this work changes the questions of nursing, then, is by introducing a dynamic relationship between the boundaries of theory and the boundaries of practice. Professional questions about the boundary of the nursing role must appeal to knowledge available to nurses at a given time. So the disciplinary expertise of nurses—nursing knowledge—is part of the identification of their professional role. But the knowledge developed by nursing research is, in turn, determined by the needs of the profession at a given time. It follows that questions about the scope of nursing knowledge and the boundaries of the nursing role are not to be answered once and for all. These issues must remain alive. Since we can expect both health care and health science to change, the scope of nursing knowledge and the nursing role must change as well. It is the ongoing responsibility of nurse scholars to be vigilant about the boundaries of their intellectual and practical discipline.

Nursing knowledge and the relevance gap

At the very outset of this work, we remarked on the simply clarity of Pamela Reed and Lisa Lawrence's definition of nursing knowledge:

> *"Nursing knowledge refers to knowledge warranted as useful and significant to nurses and patients in understanding and facilitating human health processes."* (Reed & Lawrence, 2008, p. 423)

Having explored the background issues, we now can appreciate just how radical this definition is. The warrant for nursing knowledge comes from the same kind of systematic investigation as is found in other sciences. The usefulness and significance arise from the nursing standpoint. The perspective on health provided by the nurses' role gives nursing knowledge its identity and unique character.

A potential problem with Reed and Lawrence's definition of nursing knowledge is that it makes the relevance gap seem like an illusion. By definition, nursing knowledge must be relevant to practice. Since there is plenty of research that is useful to nurses, there is no relevance gap. This "solution" to the problem of the relevance gap has the air of definitional fiat. One might argue, then, that the problem of the relevance gap has not been resolved; it has been hidden.

While there is a sense in which the relevance gap is an illusion, definitional fiat is not the solution. Nurses experience the relevance gap as a mismatch between the needs of the profession and the results of (some) nursing research. The relevance gap is a real phenomenon, but it was created by a philosophical illusion. An ideal of knowledge guided nurse scholars as they constructed their discipline. This powerful and widely shared philosophical image of knowledge was a distortion of the scientific enterprise. As a result of this false ideal, nurses sought a basic science of nursing. This project is out of touch with the needs of practice. The solution suggested here is to reconceptualize theory, method, and professional values. The new philosophical framework highlights the importance of work that is already done by nurse scholars—exactly the work that practicing nurses already find useful and important. The relevance gap is closed, not by new kinds of science, but by new kinds of philosophy.

New questions about evidence-based nursing practice

If nursing knowledge, properly construed, must be relevant to practice, it changes some of the questions that we should ask about evidence-based practice.[1] One of the issues in the literature has been to sort out the relationship between nursing expertise and research evidence (Rycroft-Malone *et al.*, 2004; Paley, 2006a). It is useful, in this discussion, to distinguish between disciplinary knowledge and clinical judgment. This essay has focused on research and theory development. Therefore, the sense of "nursing knowledge" developed here is disciplinary, not individual. Individual nurses, of course, have knowledge. A nurse's capacity for clinical judgment is the product of several different factors, one of which is the knowledge created by the nursing discipline. Clinical judgment also depends on values, both those of the nurse and of the client. Finally, clinical judgment is partly constituted by an embodied set of capacities for recognition and response. This latter component of (individual) nursing knowledge was captured by Carper's aesthetic and personal knowing patterns (Carper, 1978) as well as Benner's work on expertise (Benner, 1984). Many of the difficult questions about evidence-based practice concern the relationship of disciplinary knowledge (represented as the evidence for practice) and clinical judgment. However, because this work has concerned only disciplinary knowledge,

---

[1] Evidence-based practice is a large and complicated topic. Doing justice to all of the relevant questions—even just the philosophically interesting ones—would take another book. The discussion here is limited to a couple of areas where the questions change in the light of the philosophical positions developed above.

we must limit our discussion to the problems of evidence-based practice relevant to it.

Some of the literature on evidence-based practice goes to great length trying to ensure that nursing theories are represented in the evidence base. A good example is "On nursing theories and evidence," by Fawcett *et al.* (2001). This essay suggests that each of Carper's four patterns be regarded as a kind of theory. These nurse scholars are concerned that nursing theory be appropriately represented in the evidence base for practice; hence their call for "theory-guided, evidence-based practice." From the perspective developed in this work, we can distinguish two issues in their general concern.

First, Fawcett *et al.*, like many contributors to the evidence-based nursing practice literature, are working with the idea that nursing knowledge is unified from the top down. Unless the evidence base is explicitly linked to grand theories or conceptual models, the evidence for practice is not nursing knowledge. With respect to this issue, of course, our work has argued for a different perspective. If nursing knowledge is defined by the nursing standpoint, then there is no need to worry that, without grand theories, the nursing perspective will not be represented. Nursing knowledge *is* knowledge that responds to nursing problems. Against this background, the problems of evidence-based practice become somewhat different: How can the system be designed to (efficiently and effectively) deliver knowledge that meets nurses' needs? The evidence-based practice system was designed to serve the needs of physicians. How must it change to serve the needs of nurses? How can systems be designed that support nurse autonomy? If these questions are answered, the nursing perspective will have been represented.

The second issue is created by an ambiguity in the term "theory" that has troubled nursing for decades. Chapter 15 argued that the conceptual models of the 1950s and 1960s theorists were distorted and misrepresented by subsequent philosophical views of nursing science. These theorists were articulating models for nursing practice. They articulate a normative conception of what nursing is and should be. In this way, they are expressions of the self-understanding of nurses. These might be considered "theories of nursing," but they are not theories in the same sense that the gate-control theory of pain is a "theory." This kind of inquiry is best understood as a philosophy of nursing.

Some of the critics of evidence-based practice, such as Gail Mitchell (1999) have worried that evidence-based practice will exclude the kind of theoretical guidance most important to nurses. Once we have distinguished philosophies of nursing from empirical theories, the problem can be clearly framed. Mitchell does not doubt that empirical knowledge is important for nurses. And if nursing knowledge is defined by the nursing standpoint, then it is unproblematic to let the results of research inform practice. The concern is that appeal to clinical trials or outcome research will somehow supplant the intelligent response to nursing problems. This is primarily a concern about nurse education and management, rather than about evidence or scientific theory. The question, then, is not about whether nursing should be based on evidence, but how philosophies of nursing (conceptual models) should be integrated into nursing education and management.

New maps, new directions

The new map of nursing knowledge fundamentally changes our orientation to concepts, values, theories, and methods in nursing. It does not suggest changes in the content of nursing research, nor does it hint at new topics for investigation. Rather, as a philosophy of nursing science, this work has engaged nursing scholarship at the metatheoretical level. It has suggested new ways of thinking about scientific theory, and new ways of understanding the relationship between nursing science and professional practice. It has tried to redraw the map of the discipline.

The benefit of this new map is that it permits nurse scholars to ask different kinds of questions about their work. Those queries, this chapter has argued, are concrete and substantive, and they promote research that fills the relevance gap. Of course, whether the gap closes depends not on philosophers, but on nurse researchers. The real value of the philosophical orientation presented here, then, must be judged by the scientific consequences of the new questions. This perspective will be successful insofar as it supports a more robust science that is more useful to professional nurses. In other words, a philosophy of nursing science must be judged by its capacity to help nurse scholars create better nursing knowledge.

References

Abdellah, F. (1967) The nature of nursing science. *Nursing Research*, **18** (5), 390–393.

Ajzen, I. (1985) From intentions to actions: a theory of planned behavior. In: Kuhl, J. & Beckmann, J. (eds) *Action Control: from Cognition to Behavior*, pp. 11–39. Springer, New York.

Alexander, S.E. (1957) Nursing care of a patient after breast surgery. *The American Journal of Nursing*, **57** (12), 1571–1572.

Allen, M.N. & Jensen, L. (1990) Hermeneutical inquiry: meaning and scope. *Western Journal of Nursing Research*, **12** (2), 241–253.

Allmark, P. (1995) A classical view of the theory-practice gap in nursing. *Journal of Advanced Nursing*, **22** (1), 18–23.

American Nurses Association (2009) *Code of Ethics for Nurses (with Interpretive Statements)*. Available online at: http://nursingworld.org/ethics/code/protected_nwcoe813.htm (accessed April 19, 2009).

Anderson, E. (1995) Knowledge, human interests, and objectivity in feminist epistemology. *Philosophical Topics*, **23** (2), 27–58.

Antony, L. (1993) Quine as feminist: the radical import of naturalized epistemology. In: Antony, L. & Witt, C. (eds) *A Mind of One's Own*. Westview Press, Boulder, CO, 110–153.

Barrett, E.A.M. (2002) What is nursing science? *Nursing Science Quarterly*, **15** (1), 51–60.

Batey, M.V. (1971) Conceptualizing the research process. *Nursing Research*, **20** (4), 296–301.

Bechtel, W. (ed.) (1986) *Integrating Scientific Disciplines*. Martinus Nijhoff, Dordrecht.

Bechtel, W. & Richardson, R.C. (1993) *Discovering Complexity: Decomposition and Localization as Strategies in Scientific Research*. Princeton University Press, Princeton, NJ.

Beckstrand, J. (1978a) The notion of a practice theory and the relationship of scientific and ethical knowledge to practice. *Research in Nursing and Health*, **1** (3), 131–136.

Beckstrand, J. (1978b) The need for a practice theory as indicated by the knowledge used in the conduct of practice. *Research in Nursing and Health*, **1** (4), 175–179.

Beckstrand, J. (1980) A critique of several conceptions of practice theory in nursing. *Research in Nursing and Health*, **3** (2), 69–79.

Benner, P. (1984) *From Novice to Expert*. Addison-Wesley, Menlo Park, CA.

Bixler, G.K. (1952) What is research? *Nursing Research*, **1** (1), 7–8.

Bixler, G.K. & Bixler, R.W. (1945) The professional status of nursing. *American Journal of Nursing*, **45** (9), 730–736.

Blegen, M.A. & Tripp-Reimer, T. (1997) Implications of taxonomies for middle-range theory development. *ANS: Advances in Nursing Science*, **19** (3), 37–49.

Bogdan, R. & Taylor, S.J. (1975) *Introduction to Qualitative Research Methods: A Phenomenological Approach to the Social Sciences*. John Wiley and Sons, New York.

Boorse, C. (1977) Health as a theoretical concept. *Philosophy of Science*, **44** (4), 542–573.

Boorse, C. (1981) On the distinction between disease and illness. In: Caplan, A.L., Engelhardt, T. & McCartney, J.J. (eds) *Concepts of Health and Disease*, pp. 545–560. Addison-Wesley, Reading, MA.

Boorse, C. (1997) A rebuttal on health. In: Humber, J.M. & Almeder, R.F. (eds) *What is Disease?* pp. 1–134. Biomedical Ethics Reviews. Humana Press, Totowa, NJ.

Boyd, C.O. (2001) Philosophical foundations of qualitative research. In: Munhall, P. (ed.) *Nursing Research: A Qualitative Perspective*, 3rd edn, pp. 65–89. Jones and Bartlett Publishers, Boston, MA.

Boyd, R.N. (1991) On the current status of scientific realism. In: Boyd, R.N., Gasper, P. & Traut, J.D. (eds) *The Philosophy of Science*, pp. 195–222. MIT Press, Cambridge, MA.

Brennan, A.S. (1895) Comparative value of theory and practice in training nurses. *The Nursing Record and Hospital World*, **14**, 355.

Brody, J. (1984) A response to Dr. J. Fawcett's paper: "The Metaparadigm of Nursing: Present Status and Future Refinements". *Image—The Journal of Nursing Scholarship*, **16** (3), 87–89.

Brown, E.L. (1948) *Nursing for the Future: A Report Prepared for the National Nursing Council*. Russell Sage Foundation, New York.

Brown, M.I. (1964) Research in the development of nursing theory. *Nursing Research*, **13** (2), 109–112.

Browne, A. (2001) The influence of liberal political ideology on nursing science. *Nursing Inquiry*, **8** (2), 118–129.

Burkhart, P., Rayens, M.K., Oalkey, M., Abshire, D. & Zhang, M. (2007) Testing an intervention to promote children's adherence to asthma self-management. *Image—The Journal of Nursing Scholarship*, **39** (2), 133–140.

Butler, J. (1990) *Gender Trouble: Feminism and the Subversion of Identity*. Routledge, New York.

Carnap, R. (1962) *The Logical Foundations of Probability*, 2nd edn. University of Chicago Press, Chicago, IL.

Carper, B. (1978) Fundamental patterns of knowing in nursing. *ANS: Advances in Nursing Science*, **1** (1), 13–23.

Carr, E.C. (1996) Reflecting on clinical practice: hectoring talk or reality? *Journal of Clinical Nursing*, **5** (5), 289–295.

Cartwright, N. (1983) *How the Laws of Physics Lie*. Clarendon Press, Oxford.

Chinn, P.L. & Kramer, M.K. ([1983] 1999) *Theory and Nursing: Integrated Knowledge Development*, 5th edn. Mosby, St. Louis, MO.

Chodorow, N. (1978) *The Reproduction of Mothering: Psychoanalysis and the Sociology of Gender*. University of California Press, Berkeley, CA.

Churchman, C.W. (1956) Science and decision making. *Philosophy of Science*, **33** (3), 247–249.

Clark, A. (1998) The qualitative-quantitative debate: moving from positivism and confrontation to post-positivism and reconciliation. *Journal of Advanced Nursing*, **27**, 1242–1249.

Clarke, M. (1986) Action and reflection: practice and theory in nursing. *Journal of Advanced Nursing*, **11** (1), 3–11.

Cleland, V.S. (1967) The use of existing theories. *Nursing Research*, **16** (2), 118–121.

Clifford, J. & Marcus, G. (eds) (1986) *Writing Culture: The Poetics and Politics of Ethnography*. University of California Press, Berkeley, CA.

Cody, W.K. (1995) About all those paradigms: many in the universe, two in nursing. *Nursing Science Quarterly*, **8** (4), 144–147.

Cody, W.K. (1999) Middle-range theories: do they foster the development of nursing science? *Nursing Science Quarterly*, **12** (1), 9–14.

Cody, W.K. (2006) Preface. In: Cody, W.K. (ed.) *Philosophical and Theoretical Perspectives for Advanced Nursing Practice*, 4th edn. Jones and Bartlett Publishers, Sudbury, MA, ix–x.

Collins, P.H. (2000) *Black Feminist Thought: Knowledge, Consciousness, and the Politics of Empowerment*, 2nd edn. Routledge, London.

Collins, R. & Fielder, J. (1981) Beckstrand's concept of practice theory: a critique. *Research in Nursing and Health*, **4**, 317–321.

Committee for the Study of Nursing Education (1923) *Nursing and Nursing Education in the United States*. Macmillan, New York.

Conant, L.H. (1967a) Closing the practice–theory gap. *Nursing Outlook*, **15** (11), 37–39.

Conant, L.H. (1967b) A search for resolution of existing problems in nursing. *Nursing Research*, **16** (2), 114–117.

Coombs, M.A. (2004) *Power and Conflict between Doctors and Nurses: Breaking through the Inner Circle in Clinical Care*. Routledge, London.

Covert, E.C. (1917) Is nursing a profession? *The American Journal of Nursing*, **18** (2), 107–109.

Culver, C.M. & Gert, B. (1982) *Philosophy in Medicine*. Oxford University Press, Oxford.

Dallmayr, F.R. & McCarthy, T. (eds) (1977) *Understanding Social Inquiry*. University of Notre Dame Press, Notre Dame, IN.

Darden, L. (2006) *Reasoning in Biological Discoveries*. Cambridge University Press, Cambridge.

de Saussure, F. ([1916] 1959) *Course in General Linguistics*. Philosophical Library, New York.

Dickoff, J. & James, P. (1968) A theory of theories: a position paper. *Nursing Research*, **17** (3), 197–203.

Dickoff, J. & James, P. (1971) Clarity to what end? *Nursing Research*, **20** (6), 499–502.

Dickoff, J., James, P. & Wiedenbach, E. (1968a) Theory in a practice discipline part I: practice oriented theory. *Nursing Research*, **17** (5), 415–435.

Dickoff, J., James, P. & Wiedenbach, E. (1968b) Theory in a practice discipline part II: practice oriented research. *Nursing Research*, **17** (6), 545–554.

Doane, G.H. & Varcoe, C. (2005) Toward compassionate action: pragmatism and the inseparability of theory/practice. *ANS: Advances in Nursing Science*, **28** (1), 81–90.

Donaldson, S.K. (2000) Breakthroughs in scientific research: the discipline of nursing, 1960–1999. In: Fitzpatrick, J.J. & Goeppinger, J. (eds) *Annual Review of Nursing Research*, pp. 247–311. Springer, New York.

Donaldson, S.K. & Crowley, D.M. (1978) The discipline of nursing. *Nursing Outlook*, **26** (2), 113–120.

Draper, P. (1990) The development of theory in British nursing: current position and future prospects. *Journal of Advanced Nursing*, **15** (1), 12–15.

Duffy, M.E. (1986) Qualitative research: an approach whose time has come. *Nursing and Health Care*, **7** (5), 237–239.

Duffy, M.E. (1987a) Methodological triangulation: a vehicle for merging quantitative and qualitative research methods. *Image—The Journal of Nursing Scholarship*, **19**, 130–133.

Duffy, M.E. (1987b) Quantitative and qualitative research: antagonistic or complementary? *Nursing and Health Care*, **8**, 356–357.

Dumas, R.G. & Leonard, R.C. (1963) The effect of nursing on the incidence of postoperative vomiting. *Nursing Research*, **12** (1), 12–15.

Duncan, C., Cloutier, J.D. & Bailey, P.H. (2007) Concept analysis: the importance of differentiating the ontological focus. *Journal of Advanced Nursing*, **58** (3), 293–300.

Dupre, J. (1993) *The Disorder of Things*. Harvard University Press, Cambridge, MA.

Dzewaltowski, D.A., Noble, J.M. & Shaw, J.M. (1990) Physical activity participation: social cognitive theory versus the theories of reasoned action plan and planned behavior. *Journal of Sport and Exercise Psychology*, **12** (4), 388–405.

Ellis, R. (1968) Characteristics of significant theories. *Nursing Research*, **17** (3), 217–222.

Ellis, R. (1969) The practitioner as theorist. *American Journal of Nursing*, **69** (7), 1434–1438.

Ellis, R. (1971) Reaction to walker's article. *Nursing Research*, **20** (6), 494.

Ellis, R. (1982) Conceptual issues in nursing. *Nursing Outlook*, **30** (7), 406–410.

Fawcett, J. (1978) The relationship between theory and research: a double helix. *ANS: Advances in Nursing Science*, **1** (1), 36–39.

Fawcett, J. (1980a) A framework for analysis and evaluation of conceptual models of nursing. *Nurse Educator*, **5** (6), 10–14.

Fawcett, J. (1980b) On research and the professionalization of nursing. *Nursing Forum*, **19** (3), 310–318.

Fawcett, J. (1983) Contemporary nursing research: its relevance for practice. In: Chaska, N.L. (ed.) *The Nursing Profession: A Time to Speak*, pp. 169–181. McGraw-Hill, New York.

Fawcett, J. (1984) The metaparadigm of nursing: future status and current refinements. *Image—The Journal of Nursing Scholarship*, **16**, 84–87.

Fawcett, J. (1989) *Analysis and Evaluation of Conceptual Models of Nursing*, 2nd edn. F.A. Davis, Philadelphia.

Fawcett, J. (1993) From a plethora of paradigms to parsimony in world-views. *Nursing Science Quarterly*, **6**, 56–58.

Fawcett, J. ([1985] 1999) *The Relationship of Theory and Research*, 3rd edn. F.A. Davis Company, Philadelphia.

Fawcett, J. (2005a) *Contemporary Nursing Knowledge: Analysis and Evaluation of Nursing Models and Theories*, 2nd edn. F. A. Davis, Philadelphia.

Fawcett, J. (2005b) Criteria for evaluation of theory. *Nursing Science Quarterly*, **18** (2), 131–135.

Fawcett, J. & Alligood, M.R. (2005) Influences on advancement of nursing knowledge. *Nursing Science Quarterly*, **18** (3), 227–232.

Fawcett, J., Watson, J., Neuman, B., Walker, P. & Fitzpatrick, J. (2001) On nursing theories and evidence. *Image—The Journal of Nursing Scholarship*, **33** (2), 115–119.

Flaskerud, J.H. & Halloran, E.J. (1980) Areas of agreement in nursing theory development. *ANS: Advances in Nursing Science*, **3** (1), 1–7.

Flexner, A. ([1915] 2001) Is social work a profession? *Research on Social Work Practice*, **11** (2), 152–165.

Fodor, J.A. & Lepore, E. (1992) *Holism: A Shoppers Guide*. Blackwell, Oxford.

Folta, J.R. (1997) The author comments. In: Nicoll, L.H. (ed.) *Perspectives on Nursing Theory*, 3rd edn. Lippincott, Philadelphia, 54.

Ford-Gilboe, M., Campbell, J. & Berman, H. (1995) Stories and numbers: coexistence without compromise. *ANS: Advances in Nursing Science*, **18** (1), 14–26.

Fox Keller, E. (1978) Gender and science. *Psychoanalysis and Contemporary Thought*, **1**, 409–433.

Friesner, S.A., Curry, D.M. & Moddeman, G.R. (2006) Comparison of two pain-management strategies during chest tube removal: relaxation exercise with opioids and opioids alone. *Heart and Lung*, **35** (4), 269–276.

Gardner, G. (2006) New perspectives on old debates: re-engineering the theory practice gap. *Australian Journal of Advanced Nursing*, **24** (2), 7–8.

Garfinkel, A. (1981) *Forms of Explanation*. Yale University Press, New Haven, CT.

Geertz, C. (1973) *The Interpretation of Cultures*. Basic Books, New York.

George, J. (ed.) ([1980] 1990) *Nursing Theories: The Base for Professional Practice*, 3rd edn. Appleton & Lange, Norwalk, CT.

Giddings, L.S. & Grant, B.M. (2007) A Trojan horse for positivism? *ANS: Advances in Nursing Science*, **30** (1), 52–60.

Giere, R.N. (1988) *Explaining Science: A Cognitive Approach*. University of Chicago Press, Chicago.

Giere, R.N. (2000) Theories. In: Newton-Smith, W.H. (ed.) *A Companion to the Philosophy of Science*, pp. 515–524. Blackwell, Oxford.

Giere, R.N., Bickle, J. & Mauldin, R.F. (2006) *Understanding Scientific Reasoning*, 5th edn. Thomson Wadsworth, Belmont, CA.

Glaser, B.G. & Strauss, A.L. (1966) The purpose and credibility of qualitative research. *Nursing Research*, **15** (1), 56–61.

Good, M. & Moore, S.M. (1996) Clinical practice guidelines as a new source of middle-range theory: focus on acute pain. *Nursing Outlook*, **44** (2), 74–79.

Goodman, N. (1955) *Fact, Fiction, and Forecast*. Bobbs-Merrill Company, Indianapolis, IN.

Goodwin, L.D. & Goodwin, W.L. (1984) Qualitative vs. quantitative research or qualitative and quantitative research? *Nursing Research*, **33** (6), 378–380.

Gortner, S. (2000) Knowledge development in nursing: our historical roots and future opportunities. *Nursing Outlook*, **48** (2), 60–67.

Gortner, S.R. (1993) Nursing's syntax revisited: a critique of philosophies said to influence nursing theories. *International Journal of Nursing Studies*, **30** (6), 477–488.

Gowan, S.M.O. (1946) *Proceedings of the Workshop on Administration of Collegiate Programs in Nursing, June 12–24, 1944*. Catholic University Press of America, Washington, DC.

Gunter, L.M. (1962) Notes on a theoretical framework for nursing research. *Nursing Research*, **11** (4), 219–222.

Haack, S. (1993) Epistemological reflections of an old feminist. *Reason Papers*, **18**, 31–43.

Haase, J.E. & Myers, S.T. (1988) Reconciling paradigm assumptions of qualitative and quantitative research. *Western Journal of Nursing Research*, **10** (2), 128–137.

Hacking, I. (1983) *Representing and Intervening*. Cambridge University Press, Cambridge.

Hanson, N. (1958) *Patterns of Discovery*. Cambridge University Press, Cambridge.

Harding, S. (1991) *Whose Science? Whose Knowledge?* Cornell University Press, Ithaca, NY.

Harding, S. (1995) Strong objectivity: a response to the new objectivity question. *Synthese*, **104**, 331–339.

Harding, S. (ed.) (2003) *The Feminist Standpoint Theory Reader: Intellectual and Political Controversies*. Routledge, New York.

Hardy, M.E. ([1973] 1997) Theories: components, development, evaluation. In: Nicoll, L.H. (ed.) *Perspectives On Nursing Theory*, 3rd edn, pp. 432–442. Lippincott, Philadelphia.

Hardy, M.E. (1978) Perspectives on nursing theory. *ANS: Advances in Nursing Science*, **1** (1), 27–48.

Hartsock, N.C. (1983) The feminist standpoint: developing the ground for a specifically feminist historical materialism. In: Harding, S. & Hintikka, M.B. (eds) *Discovering Reality*, pp. 283–310. D. Ridel Publishing Company, Dordrecht.

Heath, S.T. (ed.) (1952) *The Thirteen Books of Euclid's Elements*. Encyclopedia Britannica, Chicago.

Heiderken, L. (1962) *Nursing research*—its role in research activities in nursing. *Nursing Research*, **11** (3), 140–143.

Hekman, S. (1997) Truth and method: feminist standpoint theory revisited. *Signs: Journal of Women in Culture and Society*, **22** (2), 341–365.

Hempel, C. (1965) *Aspects of Scientific Explanation and Other Essays in the Philosophy of Science*. The Free Press, New York.

Henderson, V. (1956) Research in nursing practice—when? *Nursing Research*, **4** (3), 99.

Henderson, V. (1966) *The Nature of Nursing*. The Macmillan Company, New York.

Higgins, P.A. & Moore, S.M. (2000) Levels of theoretical thinking in nursing. *Nursing Outlook*, **48** (4), 179–183.

Hilbert, H. (1959) Directions apparent in nursing research. *Nursing Research*, **8** (4), 187–188.

Hupcey, J.E. & Penrod, J. (2005) Concept analysis: examining the state of the science. *Research and Theory for Nursing Practice: An International Journal*, **19** (2), 197–208.

Hyde, E. (1922) Correlation of theory and practice in schools of nursing. *American Journal of Nursing*, **22** (9), 744–747.

Im, E.-O. (2005) Development of situation-specific theories: an integrative approach. *ANS: Advances in Nursing Science*, **28** (2), 137–151.

Im, E.-O. & Meleis, A.I. (1999) Situation-specific theories: philosophical roots, properties, and approach. *ANS: Advances in Nursing Science*, **22** (2), 11–24.

Jacobs, M.K. & Huether, S.E. (1978) Nursing science: the theory-practice linkage. *ANS: Advances in Nursing Science*, **1** (1), 63–73.

Jacox, A. (1974) Theory construction in nursing: an overview. *Nursing Research*, **23** (1), 4–13.

Jacox, A. & Suppe, F. (1990) Perspectives on the relationship of noumena and phenomena to the content of the nursing discipline. In: Fitzpatrick, J.J., England, M.C., Goodman, E. & Redmon, M. (eds) *Proceedings of the First and Second Annual Rosemary Ellis Scholars' Retreat*, pp. 283–303. Frances Payne Bolton School of Nursing of Case Western Reserve University, Cleveland, OH.

Jacox, A. & Webster, G. (1986) Competing theories of science. In: Nicoll, L.H. (ed.) *Perspectives on Nursing Theory*, pp. 423–431. Lippincott, Philadelphia.

Jeffery, R.C. (1956) Valuation and acceptance of scientific hypotheses. *Philosophy of Science*, **23** (3), 237–246.

Johnson, D. (1959a) A philosophy of nursing. *Nursing Outlook*, **7** (4), 198–200.

Johnson, D. (1959b) The nature of a science of nursing. *Nursing Outlook*, **7** (5), 291–294.

Johnson, D. (1968) Theory in nursing: borrowed and unique. *Nursing Research*, **17**(3), 206–209.

Johnson, D. (1974) Development of theory: a requisite for nursing as a primary health profession. *Nursing Research*, **23** (5), 372–377.

Johnson, J.E. (1973) Effects of accurate expectations about sensations on the sensory and distress components of pain. *Journal of Personality and Social Psychology*, **27** (2), 261–275.

Johnson, J.E. & Rice, V.H. (1974) Sensory and distress components of pain: implications for the clinical study of pain. *Nursing Research*, **23** (3), 203–209.

Johnson, J.E., Rice, V.H., Fuller, S.S. & Endress, P. (1978) Sensory information, instruction in a coping strategy, and recovery from surgery. *Research in Nursing and Health*, **1** (1), 4–17.

Johnson, J.L. & Ratner, P. (1997) The nature of the knowledge used in practice. In: Thorne, S.E. & Hayes, V.E. (eds) *Nursing Praxis: Knowledge and Action*, pp. 3–22. Sage Publications, Thousand Oaks, CA.

Kikuchi, J.F. (2003) Nursing knowledge and the problem of worldviews. *Research and Theory for Nursing Practice: An International Journal*, **17** (1), 7–17.

Kim, H.S. (1989) Theoretical thinking in nursing: problems and prospects. *Recent Advances in Nursing*, **24**, 106–122.

Kincaid, H. & McKitrick, J. (eds) (2007) *Establishing Medical Reality: Essays in the Metaphysics and Epistemology of Biomedical Science*. Springer, Dordrecht.

King, I.M. (1971) *Toward a Theory for Nursing: General Concepts of Human Behavior*. John Wiley and Sons, New York.

Kirkham, S.R. & Anderson, J. (2002) Postcolonial nursing scholarship: from epistemology to method. *ANS: Advances in Nursing Science*, **25** (1), 1–17.

Klenow, D.J. (1981) Qualitative methodology: a neglected resource in nursing research. *Research in Nursing and Health*, **4**, 281–282.

Knafl, K.A., Pettengill, M.M., Bevis, M.E. & Kirchoff, K.T. (1988) Blending qualitative and quantitative approaches to instrument development and data collection. *Journal of Professional Nursing*, **4**, 30–37.

Kripke, S.A. (1980) *Naming and Necessity*. Basil Blackwell, Oxford.

Kuhn, T. ([1962] 1970) *The Structure of Scientific Revolutions*, 2nd edn. Chicago University Press, Chicago.

Kuhn, T. (1977) Objectivity, value judgment, and theory choice. In: *The Essential Tension*, pp. 320–339. University of Chicago Press, Chicago.

Larsen, K., Adamsen, L., Bjerregaard, L. & Madsen, J.K. (2002) There is no gap 'Per Se' between theory and practice: research knowledge and clinical knowledge are developed in difference contexts and follow their own logic. *Nursing Outlook*, **50** (5), 204–212.

Lauden, L. (1977) *Progress and its Problems: Toward a Theory of Scientific Growth*. University of California Press, Berkeley, CA.

Lauden, L. (1984) *Science and Values*. University of California Press, Berkeley, CA.

Lauder, W. (1994) Beyond reflection: practical wisdom and the practical syllogism. *Nurse Education Today*, **14** (2), 91–98.

Lazarus, R.S. & Folkman, S. (1984) *Stress, Appraisal, and Coping*. Springer, New York.

Leininger, M.M. (1969) Ethnoscience: a promising research approach to improve nursing practice. *Image—The Journal of Nursing Scholarship*, **3** (1), 2–8.

Leininger, M.M. (1985) Nature, rationale, and importance of qualitative research methods. In: Leininger, M.M. (ed.) *Qualitative Research Methods in Nursing*, pp. 1–25. Grune & Stratton, New York.

Lenz, E.R., Pugh, L.C., Milligan, R.A., Gift, A.G. & Suppe, F. (1997) The middle-range theory of unpleasant symptoms: an update. *ANS: Advances in Nursing Science*, **19** (3), 14–27.

Lenz, E.R., Suppe, F., Gift, A.G., Pugh, L.C. & Milligan, R.A. (1995) Collaborative development of middle-range theories: toward a theory of unpleasant symptoms. *ANS: Advances in Nursing Science*, **17** (3), 1–13.

Levi, I. (1960) Must the scientist make value judgments? *Journal of Philosophy*, **57**, 345–457.

Liehr, P. & Smith, M.J. (1999) Middle range theory: spinning research and practice to create knowledge for the new millennium. *ANS: Advances in Nursing Science*, **21** (4), 81–91.

Lincoln, Y.S. & Guba, E.G. (1985) *Naturalistic Inquiry*. Sage Publications, Beverly Hills, CA.

Litchfield, M.C. & Jónsdóttir, H. (2008) A practice discipline that's here and now. *ANS: Advances in Nursing Science*, **31** (1), 79–91.

Longino, H. (1990) *Science as Social Knowledge: Values and Objectivity in Scientific Inquiry*. Princeton University Press, Princeton, NJ.

Makkreel, R. (1992) *Dilthey: Philosopher of the Human Studies*. Princeton University Press, Princeton, NJ.

Margolis, J. (1976) The concept of disease. *The Journal of Medicine and Philosophy*, **1** (3), 238–255.

Mason, D.J. (1999) Nursing science: who cares? *The American Journal of Nursing*, **99** (12), 7.

Masterman, M. (1970) The nature of a paradigm. In: Lakatos, I. & Musgrave, A. (eds) *Criticism and the Growth of Knowledge*, pp. 59–91. Cambridge University Press, Cambridge.

Maxwell, G. (1962) The ontological status of theoretical entities. In: Feigl, H. & Maxwell, G. (eds) *Minnesota Studies in the Philosophy of Science*, pp. 3–14. University of Minnesota Press, Minneapolis, MN.

McCorkle, R. & Quint-Benoliel, J. (1983) Symptom distress, current concerns and mood disturbance after diagnosis of life-threatening disease. *Social Science and Medicine*, **17** (7), 431–438.

McHugh, N.G., Christman, N.J. & Johnson, J.E. (1982) Preparatory information: what helps and why. *The American Journal of Nursing*, **82** (5), 780–782.

McIsaac, I. (1903) The teaching of hygiene to nurses in theory and practice. *American Journal of Nursing*, **4** (3), 184–187.

McManus, L.R. (1961) Nursing research: its evolution. *The American Journal of Nursing*, **61** (4), 76–79.

McMullin, E. (1983) Values in science. In: Asquith, P. & Nickles, T. (eds) *Proceedings of the Philosophy of Science Association 1982*, pp. 3–28. Philosophy of Science Association, East Lansing, MI.

Meleis, A.I. ([1985] 2007) *Theoretical Nursing: Development and Progress*, 4th edn. Lippincott, Williams & Wilkins, Philadelphia.

Meleis, A.I. (1987) ReVisions in knowledge development: a passion for substance. *Scholarly Inquiry for Nursing Practice: An International Journal*, **1** (1), 5–19.

Meleis, A.I. (1992) Directions for nursing theory development in the 21st century. *Nursing Science Quarterly*, **5** (3), 112–117.

Meleis, A.I. (1998) A passion for making a difference: revisions for empowerment. *Scholarly Inquiry for Nursing Practice: An International Journal*, **12** (1), 87–94.

Meleis, A.I. & Im, E.-O. (1998) Transcending marginalization in knowledge development. *Nursing Inquiry*, **6** (2), 94–102.

Melzack, R. & Wall, P.D. (1965) Pain mechanisms: a new theory. *Science*, **150**, 171–179.

Merton, R.K. (1957) *Social Theory and Social Structure*, Revised edn. Free Press, Glencoe, IL.

Miller, A. (1985) The relationship between nursing theory and nursing practice. *Journal of Advanced Nursing*, **10** (5), 417–424.

Mitchell, E.S. (1986) Multiple triangulation: a methodology for nursing science. *ANS: Advances in Nursing Science*, **8** (3), 18–26.

Mitchell, G. (1999) Evidence-based practice: critique and alternative view. *Nursing Science Quarterly*, **12** (1), 30–35.

Mitchell, G. & Pilkington, F.B. (1999) A dialogue on the comparability of research paradigms—and other theoretical things. *Nursing Science Quarterly*, **12** (4), 283–289.

Mitchell, G.J. & Cody, W.K. (1992) Nursing knowledge and human science: ontological and epistemological considerations. *Nursing Science Quarterly*, **5** (2), 54–61.

Moccia, P. (1988) A critique of compromise: beyond the methods debate. *ANS: Advances in Nursing Science*, **10**, 1–9.

Morse, J.M. (1991) Approaches to qualitative-quantitative methodological triangulation. *Nursing Research*, **40**, 120–123.

Morse, J.M. (1995) Exploring the theoretical basis of nursing knowledge using advanced techniques of concept analysis. *ANS: Advances in Nursing Science*, **17** (3), 31–46.

Morse, J.M., Bottorff, J.L. & Hutchinson, S. (1996) The paradox of comfort. *Nursing Research*, **44** (1), 14–19.

Morse, J.M. & Field, P.A. (1995) *Qualitative Research Methods for Health Professionals*, 2nd edn. Sage Publications, Thousand Oaks, CA.

Munhall, P.L. (1982) Nursing philosophy and nursing research: in apposition or opposition? *Nursing Research*, **31** (3), 176–177.

Munhall, P.L. (2001) Epistemology in nursing. In: Munhall, P. (ed.) *Nursing Research: A Qualitative Perspective*, 3rd edn, pp. 37–64. Jones and Bartlett Publishers, Boston.

Nagel, E. (1961) *The Structure of Science*. Harcourt, Brace & World, New York.

Newman, B. (1982) *The Newman Systems Model: Application to Nursing Education and Practice*. Appleton-Century-Crofts, Norwalk, CT.

Newman, M. (1972) Nursing's theoretical evolution. *Nursing Outlook*, **20** (7), 449–453.

Newman, M. (1986) *Health as Expanding Consciousness*. Mosby, St. Louis, MO.

Nightingale, F. ([1860] 1969) *Notes on Nursing: What It Is and What It Is Not*. Dover Publications, New York.

Nolan, M. & Grant, G. (1992) Mid-range theory building and the nursing theory-practice gap: a respite care case study. *Journal of Advanced Nursing*, **17** (2), 217–223.

Nordenfelt, L. (1987) *On the Nature of Health: An Action-Theoretic Approach*. D. Ridel Publishing Company, Dordrecht.

Nordenfelt, L. (2007) The concepts of health and illness revisited. *Medicine, Health Care, and Philosophy*, **10** (1), 5–10.

Norris, R. (1889) A guide to medical and surgical nursing. *The Nursing Record*, **2**, 23.

Norris, R. (1891) *Norris's Nursing Notes: Being a Manual of Medical and Surgical Information for the Use of Hospital Nurses*. Sampson Low, Marston, London.

Omery, A. (1983) Phenomenology: a method for nursing science. *ANS: Advances in Nursing Science*, **5**, 49–63.

Omery, A. & Mack, C. (1995) Phenomenology and science. In: Omery, A., Kasper, C.E. & Page, G. (eds) *In Search of Nursing Science*, pp. 139–158. Sage Publications, Thousand Oaks, CA.

Oppenheim, P. & Putnam, H. (1958) Unity of science as a working hypothesis. In: Feigl, H., Scriven, M. & Maxwell, G. (eds) *Concepts, Theories, and the Mind-Body Problem*, pp. 3–36. University of Minnesota Press, Minneapolis, MN.

Orlando, I.J. (1961) *The Dynamic Nurse-Patient Relationship: Function, Process, and Principles*. G. P. Putnam and Sons, New York.

Osborne, O.H. (1969) Anthropology and nursing: some common traditions and interests. *Nursing Research*, **18** (3), 251–255.

Ousey, K. & Gallagher, P. (2007) The theory-practice relationship in nursing: a debate. *Nurse Education in Practice*, **7** (4), 199–205.

Paley, J. (1996) How not to clarify concepts in nursing. *Journal of Advanced Nursing*, **24**, 572–578.

Paley, J. (1997) Husserl, phenomenology, and nursing. *Journal of Advanced Nursing*, **26**, 187–193.

Paley, J. (1998) Misinterpretive phenomenology: Heidegger, ontology, and nursing research. *Journal of Advanced Nursing*, **27** (4), 817–824.

Paley, J. (2006a) Evidence and expertise. *Nursing Inquiry*, **13** (2), 82–93.

Paley, J. (2006b) Book review: nursing theorists and their work, sixth edition. *Nursing Philosophy*, **7**, 275–280.

Parse, R.R. (1981) *Man–Living–Health: A Theory of Nursing*. John Wiley and Sons, New York.

Parse, R.R. (2005) Parse's criteria for evaluation of theory with a comparison of Fawcett's and Parse's approaches. *Nursing Science Quarterly*, **18** (2), 135–137.

Paterson, J. & Zderad, L. (1976) *Humanistic Nursing*. John Wiley and Sons, New York.

Patton, M. ([1980] 1990) *Qualitative Evaluation and Research Methods*. Sage, Newbury Park, CA.

Penney, W. & Warelow, P.J. (1999) Understanding the prattle of praxis. *Nursing Inquiry*, **6** (4), 259–268.

Peplau, H. (1952) *Interpersonal Relations in Nursing*. G. P. Putnam and Sons, New York.

Peterson, S. (2009) Introduction to the nature of nursing knowledge. In: Peterson, S. & Bredow, T. (eds) *Middle Range Theories: Application to Nursing Research*, pp. 3–47. Wolters Kluwer Health, Lippincott Williams & Wilkins, Philadelphia.

Peterson, S. & Bredow, T. (eds) (2008) *Middle-Range Theories: Application to Nursing Research*, 2nd edn. Lippincott Williams & Wilkins, Philadelphia.

Phillips, J.R. (1977) Nursing systems and nursing models. *Image*, **9** (1), 4–7.

Phillips, J.R. (1988a) Research blenders. *Nursing Science Quarterly*, **1** (1), 4–5.

Phillips, J.R. (1988b) Diggers of deeper holes. *Nursing Science Quarterly*, **1** (4), 149–151.

Phillips, J.R. (1995) Can researchers transcend bad science? *Nursing Science Quarterly*, **8** (4), 148–149.

Phillips, J.R. (1996) What constitutes nursing science. *Nursing Science Quarterly*, **9** (2), 48–49.

Polanyi, M. (1958) *Personal Knowledge*. Routledge and Kegan Paul, London.

Popma, A.M. (1957) Cancer of the breast. *The American Journal of Nursing*, **57** (12), 1570–1571.

Popper, S.K. (1963) *Conjectures and Refutations: The Growth of Scientific Knowledge*. Routledge and Kegan Paul, London.

Popper, S.K. (1968) *The Logic of Scientific Discovery*, 2nd edn. Harper and Row, New York.

Porter, E.J. (1989) The qualitative-quantitative dualism. *Image—The Journal of Nursing Scholarship*, **21** (2), 98–102.

Powers, B.A. (1987) Taking sides: a response to Goodwin and Goodwin. *Nursing Research*, **36** (2), 122–126.

Putnam, H. (1973) Meaning and reference. *Journal of Philosophy*, **70** (19), 699–711.

Putnam, H. (1974) The 'corroboration' of theories. In: Schilpp, P. (ed.) *The Philosophy of Karl Popper*, pp. 221–240. Open Court, La Salle, IL.

Putnam, H. (1981) *Reason, Truth, and History*. Cambridge University Press, Cambridge.

Quine, W.V.O. ([1953] 1961) Two dogmas of empiricism. In: *From a Logical Point of View*, 2nd edn, pp. 20–46. Harper and Row, New York.

Quint, J.C. (1962) Delineation of qualitative aspects of nursing care. *Nursing Research*, **11** (4), 204–206.

Quint, J.C. (1963) The impact of mastectomy. *The American Journal of Nursing*, **63** (11), 88–92.

Quint, J.C. (1967) Research—how will nursing define it? The case for theories generated from empirical data. *Nursing Research*, **16** (2), 109–114.

Racher, F.E. & Robinson, S. (2002) Are phenomenology and postpositivism strange bedfellows? *Western Journal of Nursing Research*, **25** (5), 464–481.

Ragucci, A.T. (1972) The ethnographic approach and nursing research. *Nursing Research*, **21** (6), 485–490.

Reed, P.G. (1989) Nurse theorizing as an ethical endeavor. *ANS: Advances in Nursing Science*, **11** (3), 1–9.

Reed, P.G. & Lawrence, L.A. (2008) A paradigm for the production of practice-based knowledge. *Journal of Nursing Management*, **16** (4), 422–432.

Reichenbach, H. (1951) *The Rise of Scientific Philosophy*. University of California Press, Berkeley, CA.

Reissman, L. & Roher, J.H. (eds) (1957) *Change and Dilemma in the Nursing Profession: Studies of Nursing Services in a Large General Hospital*. G. P. Putnam Sons, New York.

Riehl, J.P. & Roy, S.C. (eds) (1974) *Conceptual Models for Nursing Practice*. Appleton Century Crofts, New York.

Risjord, M. (2000) *Woodcutters and Witchcraft: Rationality and Interpretive Change in the Social Sciences*. SUNY Press, Albany, NY.

Risjord, M. (2007) Ethnography and culture. In: Turner, S. & Risjord, M. (eds) *Philosophy of Anthropology and Sociology*, pp. 399–428. Elsevier, Amsterdam.

Risjord, M. (2009) Rethinking concept analysis. *Journal of Advanced Nursing*, **65** (3), 684–691.

Risjord, M., Dunbar, S. & Moloney, M. (2002) A new foundation for methodological triangulation. *Image—The Journal of Nursing Scholarship*, **34** (3), 269–275.

Roberts, M.M. (1925) The spirit of nursing. *The American Journal of Nursing*, **25** (9), 734–739.

Rodgers, B.L. (1989) Concepts, analysis, and the development of nursing knowledge: the evolutionary cycle. *Journal of Advanced Nursing*, **14**, 330–335.

Rodgers, B.L. ([1993] 2000) Philosophical foundations of concept development. In: Rodgers, B.L. & Knafl, K.A. (eds) *Concept Development in Nursing: Foundations, Techniques, and Applications*, 2nd edn, pp. 7–38. W. B. Saunders Company, Philadelphia.

Rodgers, B.L. (2000) Concept analysis: an evolutionary view. In: Rodgers, B.L. & Knafl, K.A. (eds) *Concept Development in Nursing: Foundations, Techniques, and Applications*, 2nd edn, pp. 77–102. W. B. Saunders Company, Philadelphia.

Rogers, M. (1970) *An Introduction to the Theoretical Basis of Nursing*. F.A. Davis, Philadelphia.

Rogers, M. (1992) Nursing science and the space age. *Nursing Science Quarterly*, **5** (1), 27–34.

Rolfe, G. (1998) The theory-practice gap in nursing: from research-based practice to practitioner-based research. *Journal of Advanced Nursing*, **28** (3), 672–679.

Rosaldo, R. (1989) *Culture and Truth: The Remaking of Social Analysis*. Beacon Press, Boston.

Roy, S.C. (1976) *Introduction to Nursing: An Adaptation Model*. Prentice-Hall, Englewood Cliffs, NJ.

Rudner, R. (1953) The scientist *Qua* scientist makes value judgments. *Philosophy of Science*, **20** (1), 1–6.

Rycroft-Malone, J., Seers, K., Titchen, A., Harvey, G., Kitson, A. & McCormack, B. (2004) What counts as evidence in evidence-based practice? *Journal of Advanced Nursing*, **47** (1), 81–90.

Saunders, L. (1954) The changing role of nurses. *The American Journal of Nursing*, **54** (9), 1094–1098.

Schaffner, K.F. (1980) Theory structure in the biomedical sciences. *The Journal of Medicine and Philosophy*, **5** (1), 57–97.

Schaffner, K.F. (1993) *Discovery and Explanation in Biology and Medicine*. University of Chicago Press, Chicago.

Schlotfeld, R.M. (1960) Reflections on nursing research. *American Journal of Nursing*, **60** (4), 492–494.

Schumacker, K.L. & Gortner, S. (1992) (Mis)conceptions and reconceptions about traditional science. *ANS: Advances in Nursing Science*, **14** (4), 1–11.

Schwartz-Barcott, D., Patterson, B.J., Lusardi, P. & Farmer, B.C. (2002) From practice to theory: tightening the link via three fieldwork strategies. *Journal of Advanced Nursing*, **39** (3), 281–289.

Seedhouse, D. (2000) *Practical Nursing Philosophy: The Universal Ethical Code*. John Wiley & Sons, Ltd, Chichester.

Seedhouse, D. (2001) *Health: The Foundations for Achievement*, 2nd edn. John Wiley and Sons, London.

Sellars, W. (1963) *Science, Perception, and Reality*. Routledge and Kegan Paul, London.

Sellew, G. (1928) Correlation of theory and practice in pediatric nursing. *The American Journal of Nursing*, **28** (12), 1245–1249.

Sheldon, E.B. (1963) The use of behavioral science in nursing: an opinion. *Nursing Research*, **12** (3), 150–152.

Sheldon, E.B., Johnson, D.E. & Slusher, M.A. (1959) An experimental program in nursing research. *Nursing Research*, **8** (3), 169–171.

Silva, M.C. (1977) Philosophy, science, and theory: interrelationships and implications for nursing research. *Image—The Journal of Nursing Scholarship*, **9** (3), 59–63.

Silva, M.C. (1986) Research testing nursing theory: state of the art. *ANS: Advances in Nursing Science*, **9** (1), 1–11.

Silva, M.C. & Rothbart, D. (1984) An analysis of changing trends in philosophies of science on nursing theory development and testing. *ANS: Advances in Nursing Science*, **6** (2), 1–13.

Simon, H. (1969) *The Sciences of the Artificial*, 2nd edn. MIT Press, Cambridge, MA.

Smith, D.E. (1974) Women's perspective as a radical critique of Sociology. *Social Inquiry*, **44** (1), 7–13.

Smith, K.M. (1960) The new tomorrow in nursing: what the nurse educator sees in her crystal ball. *Nursing Outlook*, **8** (10), 547–549.

Smith, M.C. (1979) Proposed metaparadigm for nursing research and theory development: an analysis of Orem's self care theory. *Image—The Journal of Nursing Scholarship*, **11** (3), 75–79.

Smith, M.J. & Liehr, P.R. (eds) (2003) *Middle Range Theory for Nursing*, 2nd edn. Springer, New York.

Sohier, R. (1988) Multiple triangulation and contemporary nursing research. *Western Journal of Nursing Research*, **10** (6), 732–742.

Solomon, S.R. (2008) *Through a Glass Darkly: The Hidden Perspectives That Challenge and Redeem Science's Self-Conception*. PhD thesis, Emory University.

Stafford, M. (1982) Responses of clinical specialists to the unitary man framework. In: Kim, M.J. & Moritz, D.A. (eds) *Classification of Nursing Diagnosis: Proceedings of the 3rd and 4th National Conferences*, pp. 267–269. McGraw Hill, New York.

Stevenson, C. (2005) Practical inquiry/theory in nursing. *Journal of Advanced Nursing*, **50** (2), 196–203.

Sugarbaker, E.D. & Wilfley, L.E. (1950) Cancer of the breast. *The American Journal of Nursing*, **50** (6), 332–335.

Suppe, F. (ed.) (1974) *The Structure of Scientific Theories*. University of Illinois Press, Urbana, IL.

Suppe, F. (1989) *The Semantic Conception of Theories and Scientific Realism*. University of Illinois Press, Urbana, IL.

Suppe, F. (1993) Middle range theories: what they are and why nursing science needs them. In: *Proceedings of the American Nurses Association's Council of Nurse Researchers: Scientific Session*. American Nurses Association, Washington, DC.

Suppe, F. & Jacox, A.K. (1985) Philosophy of science and the development of nursing theory. In: Werley, H.H. & Fitzpatrick, J.J. (eds) *Annual Review of Nursing Research*, pp. 241–267. Springer, New York.

Swanson, J.M. & Chenitz, W.C. (1982) Why qualitative research in nursing? *Nursing Outlook*, **30** (4), 241–245.

Thagard, P. (1992) *Conceptual Revolutions*. Princeton University Press, Princeton, NJ.

Thorne, S., Canam, C., Dahinten, S., Hall, W., Henderson, A. & Kirkham, S.R. (1998) Nursing's metaparadigm concepts: disimpacting the debates. *Journal of Advanced Nursing*, **27** (6), 1257–1268.

Thorne, S., Kirkham, S.R. & Henderson, A. (1999) Ideological implications of paradigm discourse. *Nursing Inquiry*, **6** (2), 123–131.

Tinkle, M.B. & Beaton, J.L. (1983) Toward a new view of science: implications for nursing research. *ANS: Advances in Nursing Science*, **5** (2), 27–36.

Tomey, A.M. & Alligood, M.R. (eds) (1998) *Nursing Theorists and Their Work*, 4th edn. Mosby, St. Louis, MO.

Twinn, S. (2003) Status of mixed methods research in nursing. In: Tashakkori, A. & Teddlie, C. (eds) *Handbook of Mixed Methods in Social and Behavioral Research*. Sage Publications, Thousand Oaks, CA, 541–556.

Upton, D. (1999) How can we achieve evidence-based practice if we have a theory-practice gap in nursing today? *Journal of Advanced Nursing*, **29** (3), 549–555.

Uys, L.R. (1987) Foundational studies in nursing. *Journal of Advanced Nursing*, **12**, 275–280.

van Fraassen, B.C. (1980) *The Scientific Image*. Oxford University Press, Oxford.

Vicinus, M. & Nergaard, B. (eds) (1990) *Ever Yours, Florence Nightingale: Selected Letters*. Harvard University Press, Cambridge, MA.

Villarruel, A.M., Bishop, T.L., Simpson, E.M., Jemmott, L.S. & Fawcett, J. (2001) Borrowed theories, shared theories, and the advancement of nursing knowledge. *Nursing Science Quarterly*, **14** (2), 158–163.

Wald, F.S. & Leonard, R.C. (1964) Towards development of nursing practice theory. *Nursing Research*, **13** (4), 309–313.

Walker, L.O. (1971) Toward a clearer understanding of the concept of nursing theory. *Nursing Research*, **20** (5), 428–435.

Walker, L.O. ([1973] 1997) Theory, practice, and research in perspective. In: Nicoll, L.H. (ed.) *Perspectives on Nursing Theory*, 3rd edn, pp. 73–80. Lippincott, Philadelphia.

Walker, L.O. & Avant, K.C. ([1983] 2005) *Strategies for Theory Construction in Nursing*, 4th edn. Pearson Prentice Hall, Upper Saddle River, NJ.

Warms, C.A. & Schroeder, C.A. (1999) Bridging the gulf between science and action: the "New Fuzzies" of neopragmatism. *ANS: Advances in Nursing Science*, **22** (2), 1–10.

Watson, J. (1981) Nursing's scientific quest. *Nursing Outlook*, **29** (7), 413–416.

Weiss, S.J. (1995) Contemporary empiricism. In: Omery, A., Kasper, C.E. & Page, G.G. (eds) In *Search of Nursing Science*. Sage Publications, Thousand Oaks, CA, 13–26.

Whall, A.L. (1993) Lets get rid of all nursing theory. *Nursing Science Quarterly*, **6** (4), 164–165.

White, J. (1995) Patterns of knowing: review, critique, and update. *ANS: Advances in Nursing Science*, **17** (4), 73–86.

Wiedenbach, E. (1964) *Clinical Nursing: A Helping Art*. Springer, New York.

Wikipedia Contributors (2009) Carpal Tunnel, *Wikipedia, The Free Encyclopedia*. April 9, 2009 16:31 UTC. Available online at: http://en.wikipedia.org/w/index.php?title = Carpal_tunnel&oldid = 282795283 (accessed April 19, 2009).

Williams, B. (1985) *Ethics and the Limits of Philosophy*. Fontana Press, London.

Wilson, J. (1963) *Thinking with Concepts*. Cambridge University Press, Cambridge.

Wimsatt, W.C. (1972) Complexity and organization. In: Schaffner, K. & Cohen, R.S. (eds) *PSA 1972: Proceedings of the 1972 Biennial Meeting of the Philosophy of Science Association*, pp. 67–86. D. Ridel, Dordrecht.

Wimsatt, W.C. (1986) Forms of aggregativity. In: Donagan, A., Perovich, A.N. & Wedin, M.V. (eds) *Human Nature and Natural Knowledge*, pp. 259–291. D. Ridel, Dordrecht.

Wise, B.V. (2002) In their own words: the lived experience of pediatric liver transplantation. *Qualitative Health Research*, **12** (1), 74–90.

Wittgenstein, L. ([1921] 1974) *Tractatus Logico-Philosophicus*. Routledge and Kegan Paul, London.

Wittgenstein, L. (1953) *Philosophical Investigations*. Macmillan Publishing Company, New York.

Wolf, L.K. (1947) *Nursing*. Appleton-Century Co, New York.

Woodward, J. (2003) *Making Things Happen: A Theory of Causal Explanation*. Oxford University Press, Oxford.

Wylie, A. (2002) *Thinking from Things: Essays in the Philosophy of Archeology*. University of California Press, Berkeley, CA.

Yeo, M. (1989) Integration of nursing theory and nursing ethics. *ANS: Advances in Nursing Science*, **11** (3), 33–42.

Young, I.M. (1988) Five faces of oppression. *The Philosophical Forum*, **19** (4), 270–290.

Index